Table of Contents

BREAKFAST RECIPES

1-Cheese Kale Pepper Breakfast Frittata

Total Time: 2 hours 20 minutes

Serving Size: 8

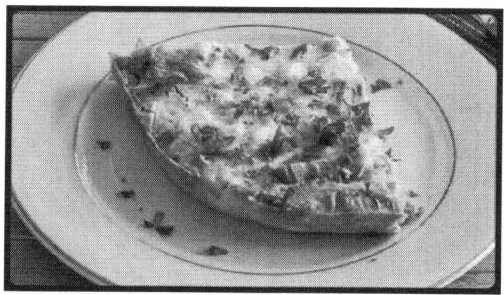

Ingredients:

- 8 eggs, beaten
- 1/2 Tsp spike seasoning
- 4 oz feta cheese, crumbled
- 1/4 cup green onion, sliced
- 6 oz red pepper, roasted and diced
- 5 oz baby kale, wash and dry
- 2 tsp olive oil

Directions:

Heat olive oil in a pan over medium-high heat.

Add kale to the pan and sauté for 4 minutes or until softened.

Spray slow cooker from inside with cooking spray.

Add cooked kale into the slow cooker.

Add green onion and red pepper into the slow cooker.

Pour beaten eggs into the slow cooker and stir well to combine.

Season with spike seasoning then sprinkle crumbled feta cheese.

Cook on low for 2 hours or until frittata is set.

Serve hot and enjoy.

Nutritional Value (Amount per Serving):

Calories 149

Fat 8.9 g

Carbohydrates 9.8 g

Sugar 5.5 g

Protein 9.1 g

Cholesterol 176 mg

2-Delicious Feta Spinach Quiche

Total Time: 7 hours 10 minutes

Serving Size: 6

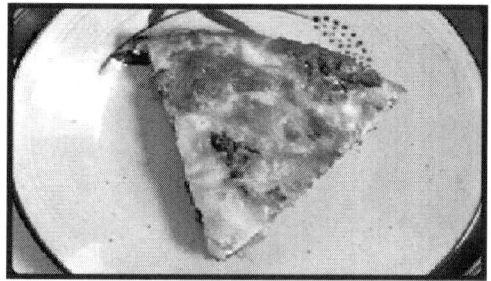

Ingredients:

- 8 eggs
- 1/4 cup cheddar cheese, shredded
- 3/4 cup feta cheese, crumbled
- 1/2 cup parmesan cheese, shredded
- 2 garlic cloves, minced
- 2 cups fresh spinach
- 2 cups almond milk
- 1/4 Tsp salt

Directions:

In a large bowl, whisk together eggs and almond milk.

Add spinach, parmesan cheese, feta cheese, garlic, and salt and stir well to combine.

Spray slow cooker from inside using cooking spray.

Pour egg mixture into the slow cooker.

Sprinkle shredded cheddar cheese over the top of egg mixture.

Cover slow cooker with lid and cook on low for 7 hours.

Nutritional Value (Amount per Serving):

Calories 367

Fat 32.5 g

Carbohydrates 6.4 g

Sugar 4 g

Protein 16.1 g

Cholesterol 247 mg

3-Easy Slow Cooker Veggie Omelet

Total Time: 1 hour 40 minutes

Serving Size: 4

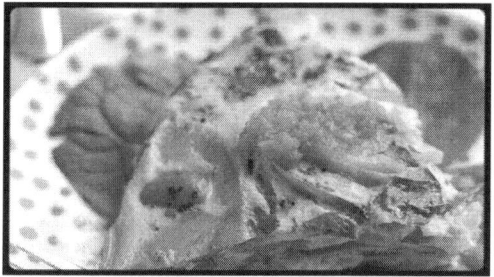

Ingredients:

- 6 eggs
- 1 tsp parsley, dried
- 1 tsp garlic powder
- 1 bell pepper, diced
- 1/2 cup onion, sliced
- 1 cup spinach
- 1/2 cup almond milk, unsweetened
- 4 egg whites
- Pepper
- Salt

Directions:

Spray slow cooker from inside using cooking spray.

In a large bowl, whisk together egg whites, eggs, parsley, garlic powder, almond milk, pepper, and salt.

Stir in bell peppers, spinach, and onion.

Pour egg mixture into the slow cooker.

Cover and cook on high for 90 minutes or until egg set.

Cut into the slices and serve.

Nutritional Value (Amount per Serving):

Calories 200

Fat 13.9 g

Carbohydrates 6.8 g

Sugar 4.1 g

Protein 13.4 g

Cholesterol 246 mg

4-Vegetable Cheese Herb Frittata

Total Time: 3 hours 10 minutes

Serving Size: 6

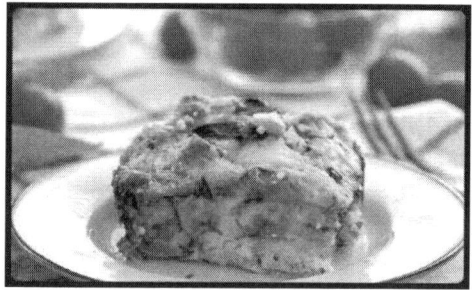

Ingredients:

- 8 eggs
- 3/4 cup goat cheese, crumbled
- 1/2 cup onion, sliced
- 1 1/2 cups red peppers, roasted and chopped
- 4 cups baby arugula
- 1 tsp oregano, dried
- 1/3 cup almond milk
- Pepper
- Salt

Directions:

Spray slow cooker from inside using cooking spray.

In a mixing bowl, whisk together eggs, oregano, and almond milk.

Season with pepper and salt.

Arrange red peppers, onion, arugula, and cheese into the slow cooker.

Pour egg mixture into the slow cooker over the vegetables.

Cover and cook on low for 3 hours.

Serve hot and enjoy.

Nutritional Value (Amount per Serving):

Calories 178

Fat 12.8 g

Carbohydrates 6 g

Sugar 3.6 g

Protein 11.4 g

Cholesterol 233 mg

5-Tasty Garlic Butter Artichokes

Total Time: 3 hours 40 minutes

Serving Size: 8

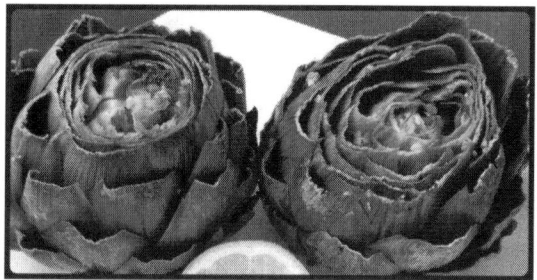

Ingredients:

- 3 medium artichokes, cut the bottom
- 1 cup water
- 1/4 cup butter
- 1/2 lemon juice
- 2 garlic cloves, minced
- Pepper
- Salt

Directions:

Cut the half inch tops of artichokes.

Place all the artichokes into the slow cooker.

Season with pepper and salt then add garlic.

Pour lemon juice over artichokes then place butter slices on top of artichokes.

Pour water into the bottom of slow cooker.

Cover slow cooker with lid and cook on high for 3 1/2 hours.

Serve hot with melted butter and enjoy.

Nutritional Value (Amount per Serving):

Calories 75

Fat 5.8 g

Carbohydrates 5.4 g

Sugar 0.6 g

Protein 1.7 g

Cholesterol 15 mg

6-Mushroom Spinach Breakfast Frittata

Total Time: 1 hour 40 minutes

Serving Size: 4

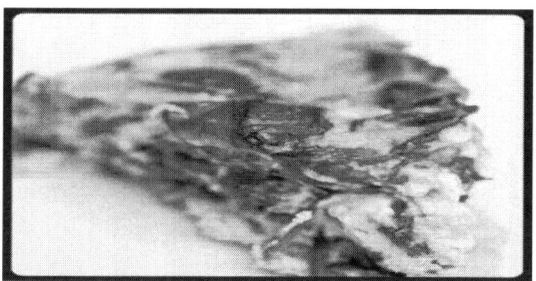

Ingredients:

- 6 eggs, beaten
- 1 cup cheese, shredded
- 1 cup fresh spinach
- 3 mushrooms, sliced
- 2 garlic cloves, minced
- Pepper
- Salt

Directions:

Spray oven-safe dish with cooking spray which fits into the slow cooker.

Combine together eggs, spinach, mushrooms, garlic, pepper, and salt into the dish.

Sprinkle cheese on top of egg mixture.

Place dish in the bottom of slow cooker.

Cover slow cooker with lid and cook on high for 90 minutes.

Cut into the slices and serve.

Nutritional Value (Amount per Serving):

Calories 215

Fat 16 g

Carbohydrates 2.1 g

Sugar 0.9 g

Protein 16.1 g

Cholesterol 275 mg

7-Healthy Zucchini Asparagus Frittata

Total Time: 1 hour 40 minutes

Serving Size: 6

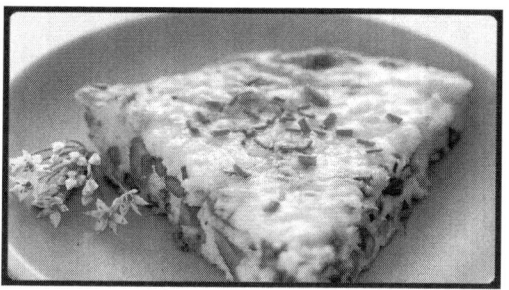

Ingredients:

- 12 eggs
- 1/4 cup fresh basil, chopped
- 1 cup parmesan cheese, grated
- 1 medium zucchini, sliced
- 8 oz asparagus, trimmed and cut into 2-inch pieces
- 2 medium shallots, chopped
- 3 tbsp olive oil
- Pepper
- Salt

Directions:

Heat olive oil in a pan over medium-high heat.

Add zucchini, asparagus, and shallots into the pan and cook until asparagus is tender.

Remove pan from heat and set aside for 10 minutes to cool.

Spray slow cooker from inside using cooking spray.

Add cooked vegetables into the slow cooker.

In a bowl, whisk together eggs, basil, parmesan, pepper, and salt.

Pour egg mixture into the slow cooker over vegetables.

Cover slow cooker with lid and cook on high for 1 hour or until frittata is set.

Cut into pieces and serve immediately.

Nutritional Value (Amount per Serving):

Calories 366

Fat 26.6 g

Carbohydrates 7.6 g

Sugar 2 g

Protein 28.6 g

Cholesterol 367 mg

8-Moist Low Carb Zucchini Bread

Total Time: 3 hours 10 minutes

Serving Size: 12

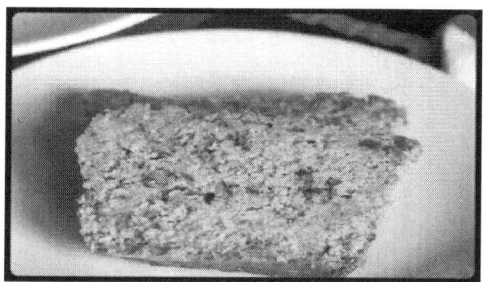

Ingredients:

- 3 eggs
- 1/2 cup walnuts, chopped
- 2 cups zucchini, shredded
- 2 tsp vanilla
- 1/2 cup pyure all purpose sweetener
- 1/3 cup coconut oil, softened
- 1/2 Tsp baking soda
- 1 1/2 Tsp baking powder
- 2 tsp cinnamon
- 1/3 cup coconut flour
- 1 cup almond flour
- 1/2 Tsp salt

Directions:

In a bowl, combine together almond flour, baking soda, baking powder, cinnamon, coconut flour, and salt. Set aside.

In another bowl, whisk together eggs, vanilla, sweetener, and oil.

Add dry mixture to the wet mixture and fold well.

Add walnut and zucchini and fold well.

Pour batter into the silicone bread pan.

Place bread pan into the slow cooker on the rack.

Cover slow cooker with lid and cook on high for 3 hours.

Cut bread loaf into the slices and serve.

Nutritional Value (Amount per Serving):

Calories 174

Fat 15.4 g

Carbohydrates 5.8 g

Sugar 1.1 g

Protein 5.3 g

Cholesterol 41 mg

9-Delicious Pecan Pumpkin Spice Cake

Total Time: 3 hours 10 minutes

Serving Size: 10

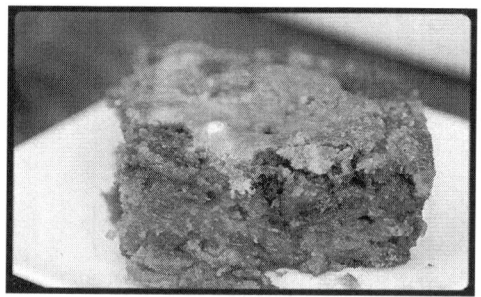

Ingredients:

- 4 eggs
- 1 tsp vanilla extract
- 1/4 cup butter, melted
- 1 cup pumpkin puree
- 1/4 Tsp ground cloves
- 1 tsp ground ginger
- 1 1/2 Tsp ground cinnamon
- 2 tsp baking powder
- 1/4 cup whey protein powder
- 1/3 cup coconut flour
- 3/4 cup Swerve sweetener
- 1 1/2 cups raw pecans

- 1/4 Tsp salt

Directions:

Spray slow cooker from inside using cooking spray.

Add pecans into the food processor and process until they resemble coarse meal.

Transfer into the mixing bowl and whisk in cloves, ginger, cinnamon, baking powder, protein powder, coconut flour, and sweetener.

Stir in eggs, vanilla, butter, and pumpkin puree until combined.

Pour batter into the slow cooker and cook on low for 3 hours.

Serve and enjoy.

Nutritional Value (Amount per Serving):

Calories 344

Fat 30.3 g

Carbohydrates 10.3 g

Sugar 2.5 g

Protein 8.2 g

Cholesterol 87 mg

10-Yummy Crust-less Cream Cheese Quiche

Total Time: 2 hours 30 minutes

Serving Size: 8

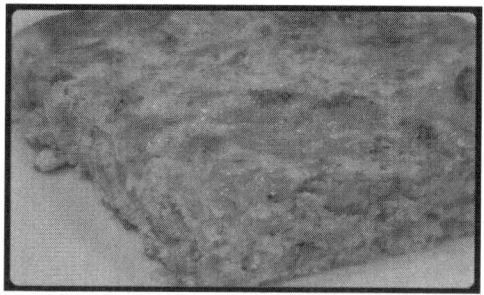

Ingredients:

- 9 eggs
- 2 cups cheese, shredded and divided
- 8 oz cream cheese
- 1/4 Tsp onion powder
- 3 cups broccoli, cut into florets
- 1/4 Tsp pepper
- 3/4 Tsp salt

Directions:

Add broccoli into the boiling water and cook for 3 minutes. Drain well and set aside to cool.

Add eggs, cream cheese, onion powder, pepper, and salt in mixing bowl and beat until well combined.

Spray slow cooker from inside using cooking spray.

Add cooked broccoli into the slow cooker then sprinkle half cup cheese.

Pour egg mixture over broccoli and cheese mixture.

Cover slow cooker and cook on high for 2 hours and 15 minutes.

Once it done then sprinkle remaining cheese and cover for 10 minutes or until cheese melted.

Serve warm and enjoy.

Nutritional Value (Amount per Serving):

Calories 296

Fat 24.3 g

Carbohydrates 3.9 g

Sugar 1.2 g

Protein 16.4 g

Cholesterol 245 mg

LUNCH RECIPES

11-Ginger Garlic Chicken

Total Time: 4 hours 10 minutes

Serving Size: 6

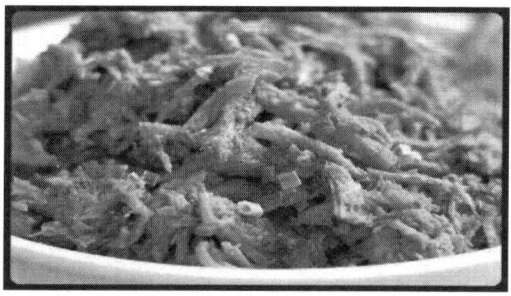

Ingredients:

- 1 1/2 lbs chicken breasts, skinless and boneless
- 1 tsp red pepper flakes
- 3 garlic cloves, minced
- 1/2 Tsp ground ginger
- 2 tbsp water
- 3 tbsp maple syrup
- 3 tbsp soy sauce
- 1/2 onion, chopped

Directions:

Place chicken into the slow cooker.

Add all remaining ingredients over the chicken,

Cover slow cooker and cook on high for 4 hours.

Using fork shred the chicken and serves.

Nutritional Value (Amount per Serving):

Calories 253

Fat 8.5 g

Carbohydrates 9 g

Sugar 6.5 g

Protein 33.6 g

Cholesterol 101 mg

12-Creamy Herb Garlic Chicken

Total Time: 4 hours 10 minutes

Serving Size: 4

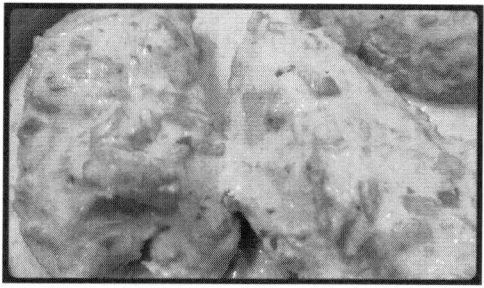

Ingredients:

- 1 lb chicken breasts, skinless and boneless
- 1/2 Tsp ground pepper
- 1 tsp oregano, dried
- 1 tsp thyme, dried
- 1 tsp rosemary, dried
- 1 tbsp garlic, minced
- 2 tbsp olive oil
- 1 tsp chicken bouillon
- 1/2 cup water
- 1/2 cup ricotta cheese
- 4 oz cream cheese

Directions:

Place chicken into the slow cooker.

Top with cream cheese and ricotta cheese.

Pour water, oregano, thyme, basil, thyme, rosemary, garlic, oil, bouillon, and pepper over the chicken.

Cover and cook on high for 4 hours.

Serve and enjoy.

Nutritional Value (Amount per Serving):

Calories 424

Fat 27.9 g

Carbohydrates 3.8 g

Sugar 0.2 g

Protein 38.7 g

Cholesterol 142 mg

13-Easy Balsamic Pot Roast

Total Time: 6 hours 10 minutes

Serving Size: 6

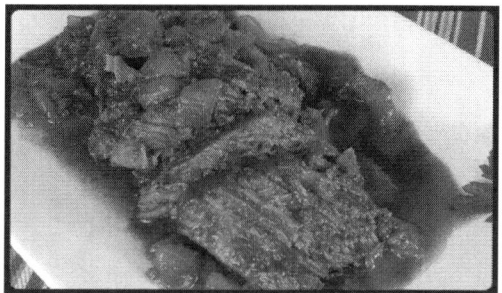

Ingredients:

- 3 lbs chuck roast, boneless
- 1/2 cup tomato sauce
- 1/2 cup balsamic vinegar
- 1 cup beef stock
- 2 large onion, sliced
- 1/4 cup water
- 2 tbsp olive oil
- 1 tbsp steak rub
- Pepper

Directions:

Rub steak seasoning and black pepper over meat.

Heat little olive oil in a pan over medium heat.

Place roast into the pan and cook until brown roast from both the sides.

Add beef stock into the saucepan and boil until sauce reduced to half then add tomato sauce and vinegar.

Add sliced onion into the slow cooker then place roast over the onions.

Pour beef stock mixture into the slow cooker.

Cover and cook on low for 6 hours.

Serve warm and enjoy.

Nutritional Value (Amount per Serving):

Calories 566

Fat 23.7 g

Carbohydrates 6.5 g

Sugar 3.1 g

Protein 76.2 g

Cholesterol 229 mg

14-Garlic and Pepper Flakes Pork Roast

Total Time: 6 hours 10 minutes

Serving Size: 8

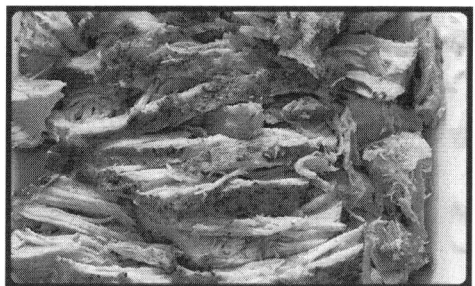

Ingredients:

- 2 lbs pork shoulder roast, boneless
- 1 tbsp maple syrup
- 1 tbsp Worcestershire sauce
- 1/3 cup balsamic vinegar
- 1/3 cup chicken broth
- 1/2 Tsp red pepper flakes
- 1/2 Tsp garlic powder
- Salt

Directions:

Season pork roast with red pepper flakes, garlic powder, and salt.

Place season pork roast into the slow cooker.

In a bowl, mix together chicken broth, Worcestershire sauce, and vinegar and pour over pork.

Add maple syrup over the pork roast.

Cover and cook on low for 6 hours.

Once pork roast is cooked then place on serving the dish and using fork shred lightly.

Pour 1/2 cup sauce over pork roast and serve.

Nutritional Value (Amount per Serving):

Calories 304

Fat 23.2 g

Carbohydrates 2.4 g

Sugar 2 g

Protein 19.3 g

Cholesterol 80 mg

15-Creamy Artichoke Spinach Dip

Total Time: 1 hour 10 minutes

Serving Size: 15

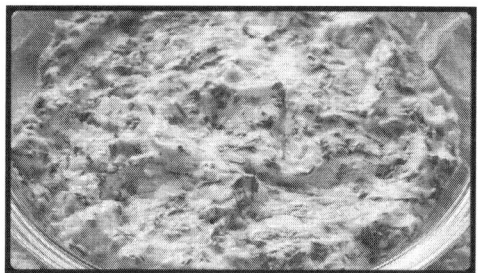

Ingredients:

- 8 oz artichoke hearts
- 1/3 cup cheese
- 1 tbsp Worcestershire sauce
- 6 oz sour cream
- 2 oz baby spinach
- 1/4 cup red onion, diced
- 1/2 cup yellow onion, diced
- 1/2 Tsp olive oil
- 1/2 Tsp pepper
- 1/4 Tsp salt

Directions:

Heat olive oil in a pan over medium heat.

Add spinach, onion, and artichoke hearts into the pan and sauté until spinach wilts. Drain excess liquid.

Transfer pan mixture into the slow cooker.

Stir in cheese, sour cream, Worcestershire sauce, pepper, and salt.

Cover slow cooker with lid and cook on low for 1 hour.

Stir well and serve.

Nutritional Value (Amount per Serving):

Calories 47

Fat 3.4 g

Carbohydrates 3 g

Sugar 0.6 g

Protein 1.7 g

Cholesterol 8 mg

16-Perfect Fresh Herb Poached Salmon

Total Time: 1 hour 25 minutes

Serving Size: 6

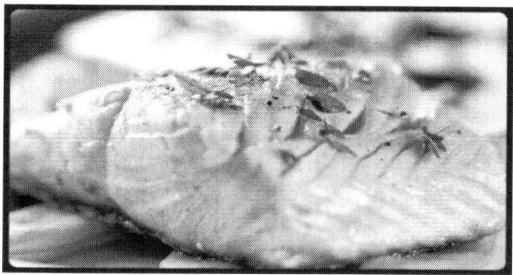

Ingredients:

- 2 lbs salmon
- 1 tsp black peppercorns
- 1 sprigs fresh tarragon
- 1 sprigs fresh dill
- 2 sprigs fresh parsley
- 1 bay leaf
- 1 shallot, sliced
- 1 lemon, sliced
- 1 cup dry white wine
- 2 cups water
- Pepper
- Salt

Directions:

Add water, peppercorns, herbs, bay leaf, shallots, lemon, wine, and salt into the slow cooker and cook on high for 30 minutes.

Season salmon with pepper and salt and place into the slow cooker.

Cover and cook on low for 45 minutes.

Serve warm and enjoy.

Nutritional Value (Amount per Serving):

Calories 243

Fat 9.4 g

Carbohydrates 3.8 g

Sugar 0.6 g

Protein 29.8 g

Cholesterol 67 mg

17-Spicy Beef Roast

Total Time: 5 hours 10 minutes

Serving Size: 6

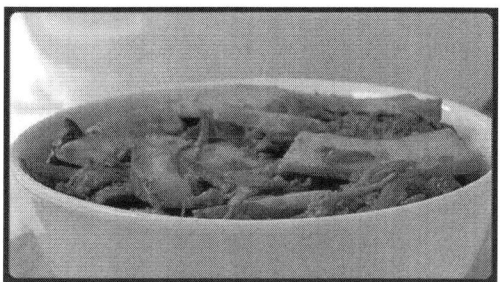

Ingredients:

- 2 1/2 lbs beef roast
- 1/4 cup coconut slices
- 1/2 Tsp ground pepper
- 1 tsp turmeric
- 2 tsp chili powder
- 1 tbsp ground coriander
- 1 tbsp meat masala
- 1 Serrano pepper, minced
- 1 tbsp ginger, grated
- 2 tbsp garlic, minced
- 2 tbsp fresh lemon juice
- 25 curry leaves
- 1 tsp mustard seeds

- 2 tbsp coconut oil
- 2 red onion, chopped
- 1 tsp salt

Directions:

Add coconut oil, mustard seeds, onion, and salt into the slow cooker and cook on high for 1 hour.

Add remaining ingredients except for coconut and cook on high for 3 hours.

Shred meat using a fork.

Add coconut slices and cook on high for 1 hour.

Serve and enjoy.

Nutritional Value (Amount per Serving):

Calories 444

Fat 18.8 g

Carbohydrates 7.5 g

Sugar 2.1 g

Protein 58.7 g

Cholesterol 169 mg

18-Spinach Lamb Curry

Total Time: 4 hours 10 minutes

Serving Size: 6

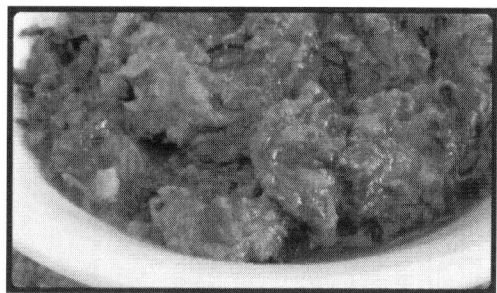

Ingredients:

- 1 lb lamb cubed
- 14 oz tomatoes, chopped
- 1 lb spinach, frozen
- 2 tsp ground cumin
- 1 tsp garam masala powder
- 1/2 Tsp chili powder
- 1 tsp turmeric powder
- 2 tsp ground coriander
- 6 whole garlic cloves
- 2 tsp cardamom
- 2 tbsp ginger, minced
- 2 garlic cloves, minced

- 1 onion, sliced

Directions:

Defrost spinach and squeeze out excess water from spinach.

Add all ingredients into the slow cooker and stir well.

Cover and cook on high for 4 hours.

Stir well and serve.

Nutritional Value (Amount per Serving):

Calories 158

Fat 6.3 g

Carbohydrates 7.7 g

Sugar 3.6 g

Protein 20.3 g

Cholesterol 68 mg

19-Delicious Pulled Pork

Total Time: 8 hours 10 minutes

Serving Size: 12

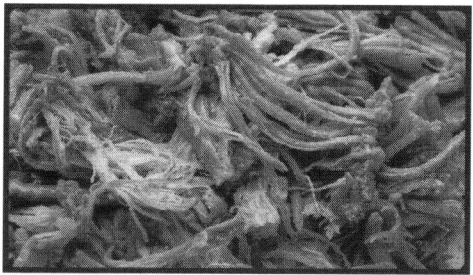

Ingredients:

- 4 lbs pork shoulder
- 3/4 cup water
- 1/4 cup apple cider vinegar
- 1 tsp onion powder
- 1 tsp garlic powder
- 1 tsp cayenne pepper
- 1 tsp pepper
- 2 tbsp paprika
- 1 tsp kosher salt

Directions:

Combine together all dried spices and rub all over pork.

Add water and vinegar into the slow cooker.

Place pork into the slow cooker.

Cover and cook on low for 8 hours.

Remove pork from slow cooker and place on serving the dish.

Using fork shred the pork.

Serve and enjoy.

Nutritional Value (Amount per Serving):

Calories 448

Fat 32.5 g

Carbohydrates 1.2 g

Sugar 0.3 g

Protein 35.5 g

Cholesterol 136 mg

20-Tasty Pork Carnitas

Total Time: 6 hours 10 minutes

Serving Size: 6

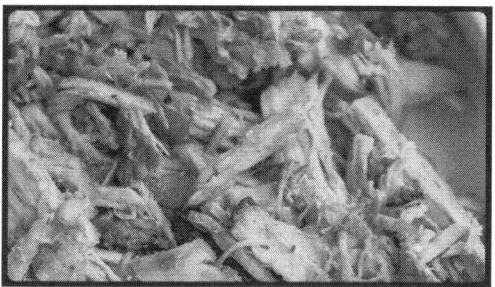

Ingredients:

- 2 lbs pork tenderloin
- 1 orange juice
- 1 lime juice
- 1 jalapeno, chopped
- 3 garlic cloves, minced
- 1/2 onion, chopped
- 1 tbsp olive oil
- 2 tsp ground cumin
- 1 tbsp oregano, dried

Directions:

Combine together olive oil, ground cumin, and oregano and rub over pork tenderloin.

Place tenderloin into the slow cooker.

Top with all remaining ingredients.

Cover and cook on low for 6 hours.

Transfer pork tenderloin on serving the dish and using fork shred the meat.

Serve and enjoy.

Nutritional Value (Amount per Serving):

Calories 256

Fat 7.9 g

Carbohydrates 4.4 g

Sugar 1.9 g

Protein 40.1 g

Cholesterol 110 mg

21-4 Ingredients Salsa

Total Time: 5 hours 5 minutes

Serving Size: 10

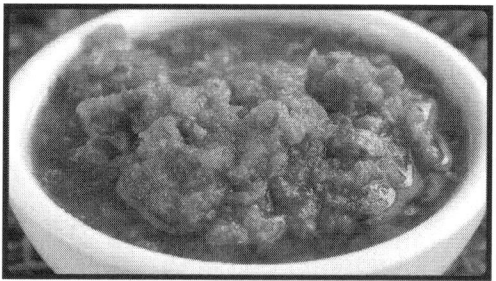

Ingredients:

- 2 jalapenos, diced
- 1 onion, sliced
- 4 cups grape tomatoes, halved
- 1/8 Tsp salt

Directions:

Add all ingredients into the slow cooker and stir well.

Cover and cook on low for 5 hours.

Smash tomatoes lightly and stir well.

Serve and enjoy.

Nutritional Value (Amount per Serving):

Calories 18

Fat 0.2 g

Carbohydrates 4 g

Sugar 2.5 g

Protein 0.8 g

Cholesterol 0 mg

22-Spinach Broccoli Dip

Total Time: 1 hour 10 minutes

Serving Size: 15

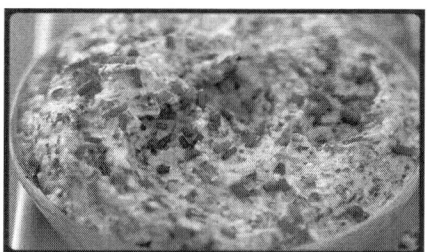

Ingredients:

- 4 cups broccoli florets, steamed
- 2 tbsp fresh lemon juice
- 1/4 Tsp black pepper
- 1 cup plain yogurt
- 1/2 tbsp capers
- 1 tbsp Worcestershire sauce
- 1 jalapeno, remove seeds and stem
- 1 shallot
- 1 cup fresh spinach

Directions:

Add broccoli, capers, Worcestershire sauce, jalapeno, shallot, and spinach into the food processor and process until mixture is smooth.

Add lemon juice, pepper, and yogurt and process until smooth.

Pour mixture broccoli mixture into the slow cooker.

Cover slow cooker with lid and cook on low for 1 hour.

Nutritional Value (Amount per Serving):

Calories 25

Fat 0.3 g

Carbohydrates 3.7 g

Sugar 1.8 g

Protein 1.8 g

Cholesterol 1 mg

23-Olive Sun Dried Tomatoes Pot Roast

Total Time: 7 hours 20 minutes

Serving Size: 6

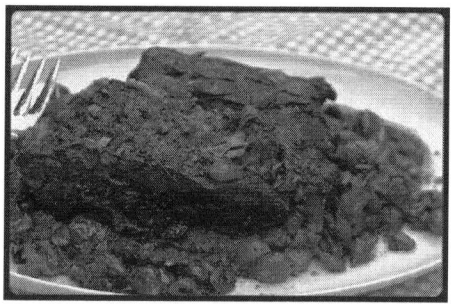

Ingredients:

- 3 lbs beef chuck roast

- 8 green olives, sliced

- 1 tsp arrowroot

- 1/4 Tsp black pepper

- 1 tsp Italian seasoning, dried

- 2 tbsp balsamic vinegar

- 1/2 cup dry red wine

- 1/4 cup sun-dried tomatoes, chopped

- 20 garlic cloves, peeled and sliced

Directions:

Add sliced garlic and sun dried tomatoes into the slow cooker.

Place beef over the garlic and tomatoes.

Pour vinegar and red wine over meat.

Sprinkle with black pepper and Italian seasoning.

Cover and cook on low for 7 hours.

Transfer meat on a platter.

Set slow cooker on high.

In a small bowl, whisk together 2 tsp water and arrowroot

and pour into the slow cooker. Stir well.

Cover and cook for another 10 minutes or until sauce thicken.

Pour sauce over meat and stir in olives.

Serve and enjoy.

Nutritional Value (Amount per Serving):

Calories 870

Fat 64.1 g

Carbohydrates 5.1 g

Sugar 0.6 g

Protein 60.2 g

Cholesterol 234 mg

24-Basil Tomato Dip

Total Time: 1 hour 10 minutes

Serving Size: 20

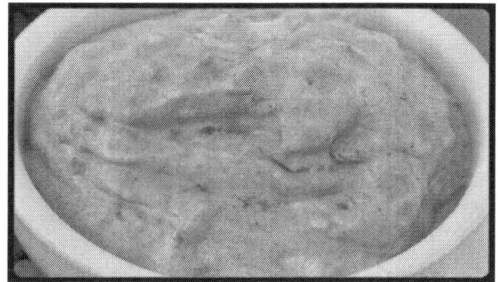

Ingredients:

- 8 oz cream cheese
- 1/4 cup sun dried tomatoes
- 1/4 Tsp white pepper
- 1 tsp pine nuts, toasted
- 3/4 oz fresh basil
- 1 tbsp mayonnaise
- 2 garlic cloves

Directions:

Add all ingredients into the slow cooker and process until smooth.

Pour mixture into the slow cooker.

Cover and cook on low for 1 hour.

Stir well and serve.

Nutritional Value (Amount per Serving):

Calories 47

Fat 4.5 g

Carbohydrates 1 g

Sugar 0.1 g

Protein 1 g

Cholesterol 13 mg

25-Dill Butter Carrots

Total Time: 2 hours 5 minutes

Serving Size: 6

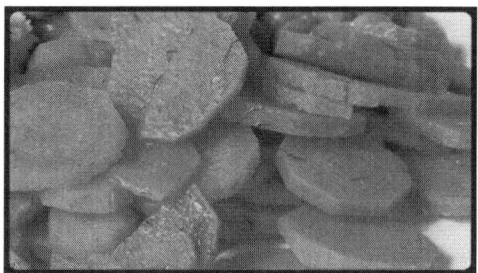

Ingredients:

- 1 lb carrots, cut into round pieces
- 3 tbsp water
- 1/2 Tsp butter
- 1 tbsp fresh dill, minced

Directions:

Add all ingredients into the slow cooker and mix well.

Cover and cook on low for 2 hours or until tender.

Stir well and serve.

Nutritional Value (Amount per Serving):

Calories 35

Fat 0.3 g

Carbohydrates 7.7 g

Sugar 3.7 g

Protein 0.7 g

Cholesterol 1 mg

26-Thyme Lemon Green Beans

Total Time: 1 hour 40 minutes

Serving Size: 4

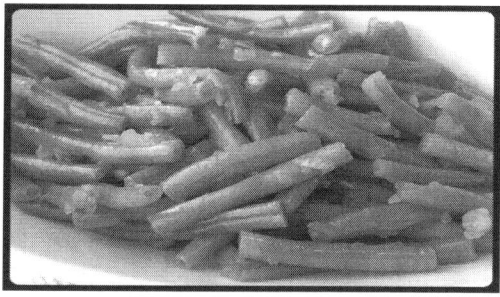

Ingredients:

- 1 lb green beans
- 2 tbsp water
- 2 tbsp fresh lemon juice
- 1 tsp fresh thyme, minced
- 1 tbsp rosemary, minced

Directions:

Add all ingredients into the slow cooker and mix well.

Cover and cook on low for 1 1/2 hours or until beans are tender.

Stir well and serve.

Nutritional Value (Amount per Serving):

Calories 40

Fat 0.4 g

Carbohydrates 8.9 g

Sugar 1.8 g

Protein 2.2 g

Cholesterol 0 mg

27-Stewed Onion Okra

Total Time: 2 hours 10 minutes

Serving Size: 4

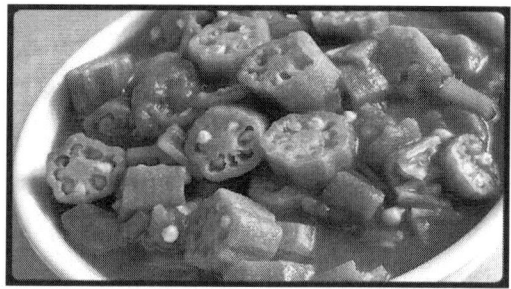

Ingredients:

- 1 1/2 cups okra, diced
- 1 tsp hot sauce
- 2 garlic cloves, minced
- 1 small onion, diced
- 2 large tomatoes, diced

Directions:

Add all ingredients into the slow cooker and stir well.

Cover and cook on low for 2 hours.

Stir well and serve.

Nutritional Value (Amount per Serving):

Calories 41

Fat 0.3 g

Carbohydrates 8.5 g

Sugar 3.7 g

Protein 1.8 g

Cholesterol 0 mg

28-Easy Lime Ginger Salmon

Total Time: 3 hours 10 minutes

Serving Size: 12

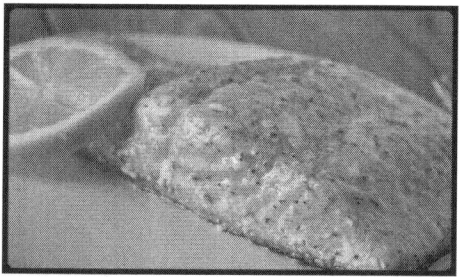

Ingredients:

- 3 lbs salmon fillet, remove bones
- 1 onion, sliced
- 1 lime, sliced
- 1/4 cup lime juice
- 1/4 cup fresh ginger, minced

Directions:

Place salmon skin side down into the slow cooker.

Pour lime juice over the salmon then add ginger.

Arrange lime and onion slices over the salmon.

Cover and cook on low for 3 hours.

Serve and enjoy.

Nutritional Value (Amount per Serving):

Calories 166   Fat 7.2 g

Carbohydrates 4.1 g

Sugar 0.8 g

Protein 22.4 g

Cholesterol 50 mg

29-Cheese Stuffed Mushrooms

Total Time: 2 hours 10 minutes

Serving Size: 4

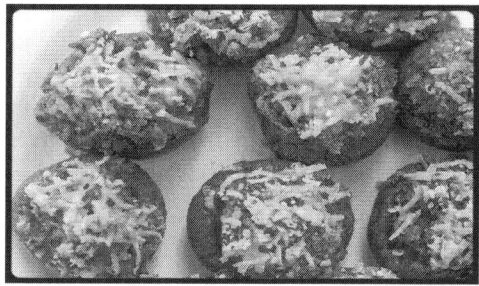

Ingredients:

- 10 large mushrooms, remove stems and diced stems
- 1/4 cup Monterey Jack cheese, shredded
- 1/8 Tsp cayenne pepper
- 1/8 Tsp pepper
- 1 tbsp olive oil
- 1/4 Tsp garlic, minced
- 1/8 Tsp salt

Directions:

Heat olive oil in a pan over medium heat.

Add garlic and diced mushroom stems into the pan and

sautés until softened.

Remove pan from heat.

Add cheese and seasoning and stir well.

Stuff pan mixture into the mushroom shells and place into the slow cooker.

Cover slow cooker with lid and cook on low for 2 hours.

Serve and enjoy.

Nutritional Value (Amount per Serving):

Calories 69

Fat 5.8 g

Carbohydrates 2.1 g

Sugar 1 g

Protein 3.6 g

Cholesterol 6 mg

30-Sesame Bell Pepper Broccoli

Total Time: 4 hours 10 minutes

Serving Size: 8

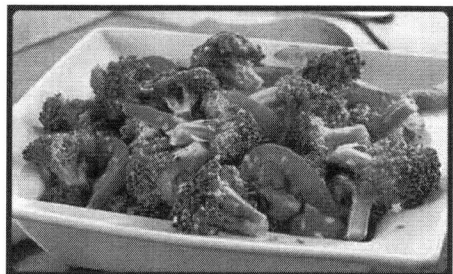

Ingredients:

- 2 lbs fresh broccoli, trimmed and cut into pieces
- 1 tbsp sesame seeds
- 4 tbsp soy sauce
- 1 onion, sliced
- 1 bell pepper, sliced
- 1 garlic clove, minced
- 1/8 Tsp pepper
- 1/2 Tsp salt

Directions:

Add all ingredients except sesame seeds into the slow cooker and stir well.

Cover slow cooker with lid and cook on low for 4 hours.

Stir well and sprinkle with sesame seeds.

Serve warm and enjoy.

Nutritional Value (Amount per Serving):

Calories 60

Fat 1 g

Carbohydrates 11 g

Sugar 3.4 g

Protein 4.2 g

Cholesterol 0 mg

DINNER RECIPES

31-Basil Thyme Beef Roast

Total Time: 8 hours 10 minutes

Serving Size: 8

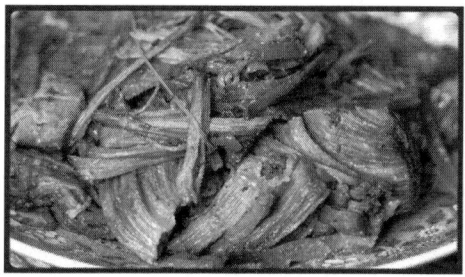

Ingredients:

- 2 1/2 lbs beef round roast
- 1/2 Tsp marjoram
- 1/2 Tsp thyme
- 1 tsp basil
- 1/2 cup red wine
- 1/2 cup water
- 1 small onion, sliced
- 1/4 Tsp pepper
- 1 tsp kosher salt

Directions:

In a small bowl, combine together all spices. Set aside.

Place beef roast into the slow cooker.

Sprinkle spice mixture over roast and top with onion.

Pour water and wine into the slow cooker.

Cover and cook on low for 8 hours.

Once beef is cooked then using fork shred the meat.

Serve and enjoy.

Nutritional Value (Amount per Serving):

Calories 281

Fat 11 g

Carbohydrates 1.3 g

Sugar 0.5 g

Protein 39 g

Cholesterol 122 mg

32-Garlic Onion Brisket

Total Time: 6 hours 30 minutes

Serving Size: 6

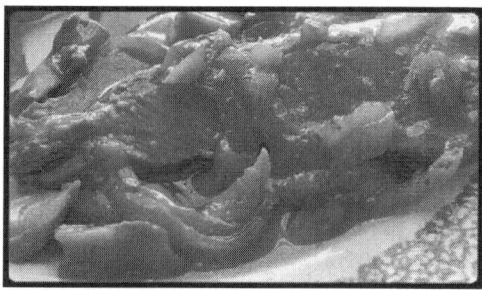

Ingredients:

- 3 1/2 lbs beef brisket
- 1 tbsp soy sauce
- 2 tbsp Worcestershire sauce
- 2 cups beef broth
- 2 large onion, sliced
- 1 tbsp olive oil
- 6 garlic cloves, minced
- Pepper
- Salt

Directions:

Heat olive oil in the pan over medium heat.

Add onion into the pan and cook until lightly caramelized about 20 minutes.

Season brisket with pepper and salt.

Heat another pan over medium heat.

Place brisket on the pan and cook until brisket appears golden brown crust.

Place brisket into the slow cooker.

Sprinkle garlic over brisket then place caramelized onion over the brisket.

Combine together soy sauce and Worcestershire sauce and pour over the brisket.

Cover slow cooker with lid and cook on low for 6 hours or until brisket is tender.

Sliced brisket and serve.

Nutritional Value (Amount per Serving):

Calories 555

Fat 19.4 g

Carbohydrates 7.2 g

Sugar 3.4 g

Protein 82.8 g

Cholesterol 236 mg

33-Spicy Coconut Chicken

Total Time: 6 hours 10 minutes

Serving Size: 5

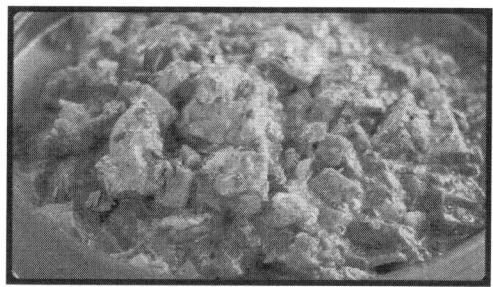

Ingredients:

- 1 lb chicken thighs, boneless and skinless

- 1 cup coconut milk

- 1 cup heavy cream

- 10 oz tomatoes, diced

- 2 tsp paprika

- 5 tsp garam masala

- 3 tbsp tomato paste

- 1 tbsp ginger, grated

- 3 garlic cloves, minced

- 2 tsp onion powder

- 2 tbsp olive oil

- 1 tsp guar gum

Directions:

Cut chicken into the pieces and add in the slow cooker.

Add grated ginger over the chicken then add all spices.

Add tomatoes, tomato paste, and olive oil. Mix well.

Add half cup coconut milk and stir well.

Cover slow cooker with lid and cook on low for 6 hours.

Once the chicken is cooked then add heavy cream, guar gum, and remaining coconut milk and stir well.

Serve and enjoy.

Nutritional Value (Amount per Serving):

Calories 444

Fat 33 g

Carbohydrates 10 g

Sugar 4.8 g

Protein 29.2 g

Cholesterol 114 mg

34-Creamy Chicken Curry

Total Time: 4 hours 10 minutes

Serving Size: 6

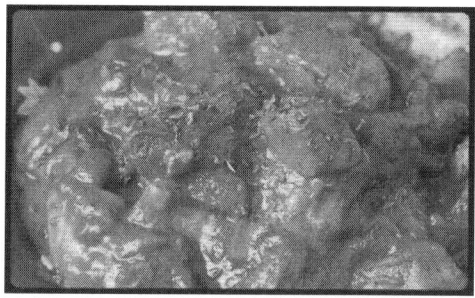

Ingredients:

- 2 lbs chicken breasts cut into pieces
- 2 tbsp arrowroot powder
- 1 tsp chili powder
- 1 tsp curry powder
- 2 tsp garam masala
- 6 oz tomato paste
- 13 oz coconut milk
- 1 medium onion, chopped
- 3 garlic cloves, minced
- 2 tbsp coconut oil
- 1/4 Tsp black pepper
- 1 tsp sea salt

Directions:

Heat coconut oil in a pan over medium heat.

Add garlic and onion to the pan and sauté for 5 minutes.

Add chili powder, curry powder, and garam masala and stir for 1 minute.

Stir in tomato paste, coconut milk, pepper, and salt.

In a small bowl, combine together 4 tbsp water and arrowroot powder and stir in coconut milk mixture. Remove pan from heat.

Add chicken into the slow cooker then pour pan mixture over the chicken.

Cover slow cooker with lid and cook on low for 4 hours.

Stir well and serve.

Nutritional Value (Amount per Serving):

Calories 508

Fat 30.7 g

Carbohydrates 12 g

Sugar 6.3 g

Protein 46.8 g

Cholesterol 135 mg

35-Spicy Pork Adobo

Total Time: 8 hours 10 minutes

Serving Size: 8

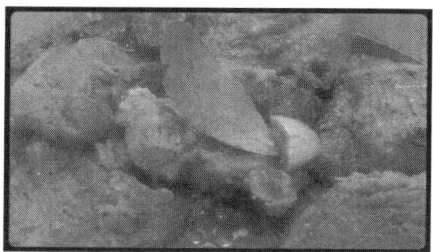

Ingredients:

- 3 lbs lean pork shoulder, trimmed
- 1/4 cup cilantro
- 2 bay leaves
- 1 tsp oregano, dried
- 1 tbsp coriander
- 1 tsp cumin
- 1 onion, chopped
- 5 garlic cloves
- 2 chipotle peppers
- 2 Ancho chili peppers, dried
- Pepper
- Salt

Directions:

In a pan, roast ancho chili peppers for 3 minutes. Set aside to cool.

Once chili is cool then remove stem and seeds.

Add chili in a small bowl and cover with water.

Add chilies in a small pot and bring to boil and simmer for 5 minutes.

Turn off the heat and set aside chili pot for 30 minutes.

Add onion, oregano, garlic, coriander, cumin, chipotles and chili pepper with 1 cup cooking liquid into the blender and blend until well combined.

Season pork shoulder with pepper and salt.

Pour little onion mixture into the slow cooker then place pork shoulder and then pour remaining onion mixture over pork.

Cover and cook on low for 8 hours.

Using fork shred the meat and serves.

Nutritional Value (Amount per Serving):

Calories 408

Fat 23.3 g

Carbohydrates 3.6 g

Sugar 1.2 g

Protein 43.8 g   Cholesterol 153 mg

36-Classic Stuffed Peppers

Total Time: 4 hours 10 minutes

Serving Size: 1

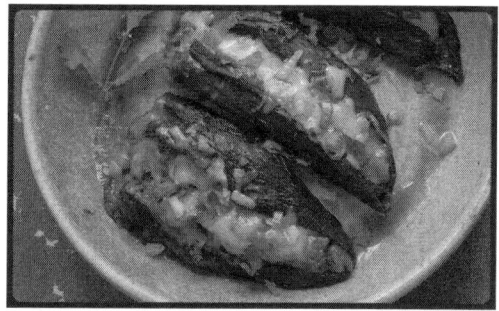

Ingredients:

- 1 Poblano pepper, cut into the half and remove seeds
- 3 tbsp tomato sauce
- 1 tbsp onion, chopped
- 1/3 lb ground beef
- 1/3 cup cauliflower, chopped

Directions:

In a pan, Add onion, and ground beef and cook until brown.

Add tomato sauce and cauliflower into the beef mixture and stir well.

Stuff mixture into the pepper halves.

Add 1/2 inch water into the slow cooker.

Carefully place stuffed peppers into the slow cooker.

Cover and cook on low for 4 hours.

Serve warm and enjoy.

Nutritional Value (Amount per Serving):

Calories 322

Fat 9.6 g

Carbohydrates 9 g

Sugar 5 g

Protein 48.2 g

Cholesterol 135 mg

37-Slow Cooker Onion Pork Chops

Total Time: 6 hours 10 minutes

Serving Size: 4

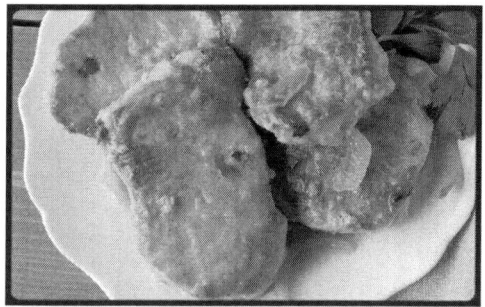

Ingredients:

- 4 loin chops, lean
- 1 tsp butter
- 2 medium onions, sliced
- 1 tsp spices mix
- Pepper
- Salt

Directions:

Add sliced onion into the slow cooker.

Place pork chops over the sliced onion and sprinkle with spice mix, pepper, and salt.

Add butter on top.

Cover slow cooker with lid and cook on low for 6 hours.

Serve and enjoy.

Nutritional Value (Amount per Serving):

Calories 287

Fat 20.9 g

Carbohydrates 5.2 g

Sugar 2.3 g

Protein 18.6 g

Cholesterol 71 mg

38-Garlic Smoked Paprika Shrimp

Total Time: 1 hour

Serving Size: 8

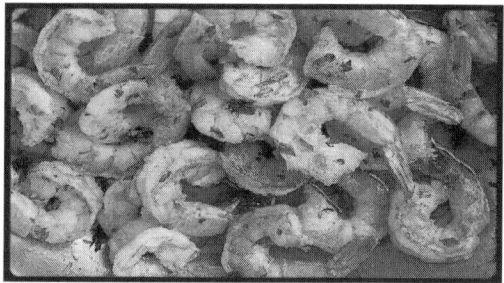

Ingredients:

- 2 lbs raw shrimp, peeled and deveined
- 1/4 Tsp red pepper flakes, crushed
- 1/4 Tsp ground black pepper
- 1 tsp paprika
- 6 garlic cloves, sliced
- 3/4 cup olive oil
- 1 tsp kosher salt

Directions:

Combine together oil, red pepper flakes, black pepper, paprika, garlic, and salt into the slow cooker.

Cover and cook on high for 30 minutes.

Add shrimp and stir well.

Cover and cook on high for 10 minutes.

Open the lid and stir again. Cover and cook for another 10 minutes.

Serve warm and enjoy.

Nutritional Value (Amount per Serving):

Calories 301

Fat 20 g

Carbohydrates 2.7 g

Sugar 0.1 g

Protein 26 g

Cholesterol 239 mg

39-Tasty Herb Bacon Chicken

Total Time: 8 hours 10 minutes

Serving Size: 4

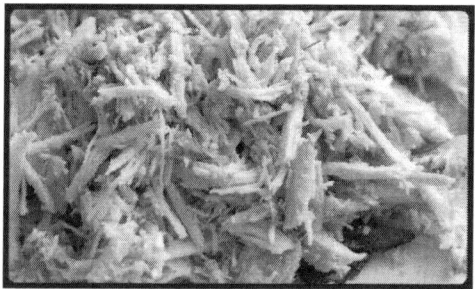

Ingredients:

- 5 chicken breasts
- 5 tbsp olive oil
- 1 tbsp rosemary, dried
- 1 tbsp oregano, dried
- 2 tbsp thyme, dried
- 10 bacon slices
- 1 tbsp salt

Directions:

Add all ingredients into the slow cooker and mix well.

Cover and cook on low for 8 hours.

Using fork shred the chicken and serves.

Nutritional Value (Amount per Serving):

Calories 619

Fat 28.6 g

Carbohydrates 2.1 g

Sugar 0.1 g

Protein 55.3 g

Cholesterol 146 mg

40-Delicious Pulled Pork Tacos

Total Time: 8 hours 10 minutes

Serving Size: 10

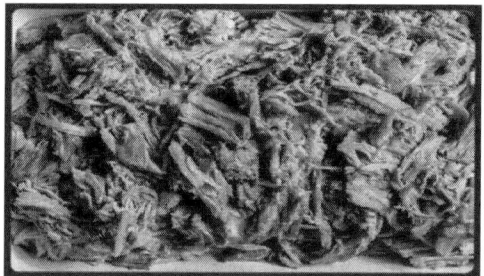

Ingredients:

- 4 1/3 lbs pork shoulder

- 1 bay leaf

- 1/2 cup beef stock

- 1/4 Tsp red pepper flakes, crushed

- 1/2 Tsp ground oregano

- 1 1/2 Tsp ground cumin

- 2 tbsp chili powder

- 1/8 Tsp ground cloves

- 1 tbsp kosher salt

Directions:

In a bowl, combine together chili powder, cloves, red pepper flakes, oregano, cumin, and salt.

Rub spice mixture all over pork.

Place pork in the refrigerator and let marinate for 2 hours.

Place marinated pork in the slow cooker with bay leaf and beef stock.

Cook on low for 8 hours.

Using fork shred the meat and serves.

Nutritional Value (Amount per Serving):

Calories 581

Fat 42.4 g

Carbohydrates 1.1 g

Sugar 0.1 g

Protein 46.2 g

Cholesterol 177 mg

41-Gluten Free Chile Verde

Total Time: 6 hours 10 minutes

Serving Size: 9

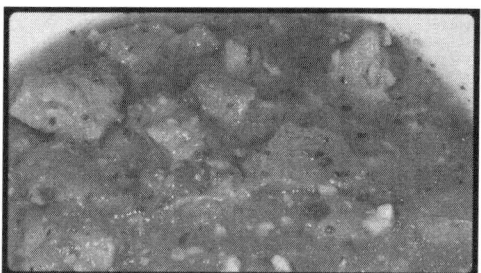

Ingredients:

- 2 lbs pork stewing meat, boneless and chopped
- 5 garlic cloves, minced
- 1 1/2 cups salsa
- 3 tbsp cilantro, chopped
- 3 tbsp butter
- 1/4 Tsp sea salt

Directions:

Set slow cooker on high and add 2 tbsp butter in slow cooker.

Once butter is melted then add 4 garlic and 2 tbsp cilantro and stir well.

Melt remaining 1 tbsp butter in a pan over medium high heat.

Add remaining garlic and cilantro into the pan and stir well.

Add chopped pork into the pan and cooked until pork is brown from all the sides.

Add pork and garlic cilantro mixture into the slow cooker.

Add salad into the slow cooker and stir well.

Cover slow cooker with lid and cook on low for 6 hours.

Serve and enjoy.

Nutritional Value (Amount per Serving):

Calories 262

Fat 13.7 g

Carbohydrates 3.3 g

Sugar 1.4 g

Protein 30.3 g

Cholesterol 97 mg

42-Healthy Brussels sprouts

Total Time: 4 hours 10 minutes

Serving Size: 8

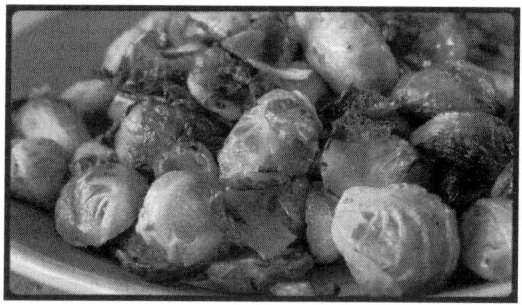

Ingredients:

- 2 lbs Brussels sprouts, rinsed and halved
- 2 tbsp olive oil
- 1/2 cup balsamic vinegar
- Pepper
- Salt

Directions:

Add olive oil and Brussels sprouts into the slow cooker.

Season with pepper and salt.

Cover slow cooker and cook on low for 4 hours.

Once Brussels sprouts are ready then drizzle with vinegar and serve.

Nutritional Value (Amount per Serving):

Calories 82

Fat 3.9 g

Carbohydrates 10.5 g

Sugar 2.5 g

Protein 3.9 g

Cholesterol 0 mg

43-Coconut Green Curry Wings

Total Time: 6 hours 10 minutes

Serving Size: 6

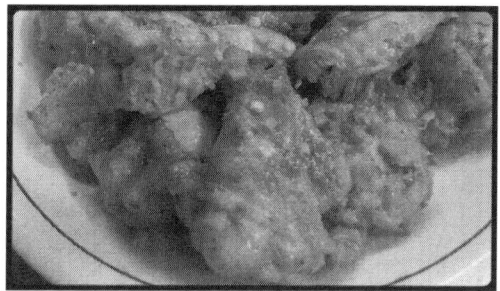

Ingredients:

- 3 lbs chicken wings
- 1 tbsp fresh cilantro, minced
- 1 tbsp fresh ginger, minced
- 1 tbsp coconut milk
- 2 oz Thai basil, minced
- 8 oz green curry paste

Directions:

Add chicken wings into the slow cooker.

In a bowl, whisk together coconut milk, cilantro, ginger, basil, and curry paste.

Pour coconut milk mixture over chicken wings and toss well.

Cover and cook on low for 6 hours.

Stir well and serve.

Nutritional Value (Amount per Serving):

Calories 322

Fat 14.3 g

Carbohydrates 6.3 g

Sugar 0.1 g

Protein 39.6 g

Cholesterol 121 mg

44-Lemon Garlic Eggplant

Total Time: 2 hours 5 minutes

Serving Size: 12

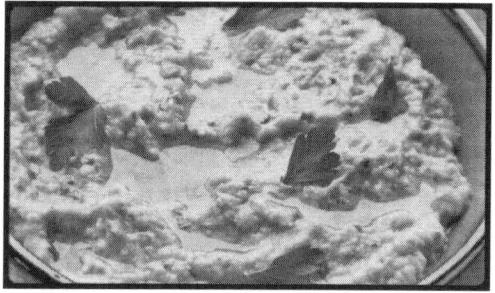

Ingredients:

- 1 lb eggplant, pierce with fork
- 2 garlic cloves
- 2 tbsp lemon juice
- 2 tbsp tahini

Directions:

Add eggplant into the slow cooker and cook for 2 hours.

Once it cooks then peels off the skin.

Slice eggplant into the half and remove seeds.

Add pulp into the food processor with remaining ingredients and process until smooth.

Serve and enjoy.

Nutritional Value (Amount per Serving):

Calories 26

Fat 1.4 g

Carbohydrates 3 g

Sugar 1.2 g

Protein 0.9 g

Cholesterol 0 mg

45-Creamy Artichoke and Shrimp Dip

Total Time: 50 minutes

Serving Size: 20

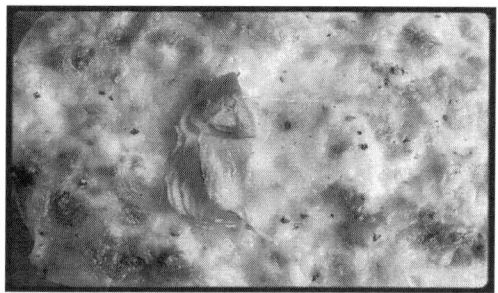

Ingredients:

- 8 oz salad shrimp, peeled
- 12 oz artichoke hearts, frozen and defrosted
- 1 1/2 Tsp old bay seasoning
- 1 tbsp Worcestershire sauce
- 1/2 cup green onion, diced
- 1/2 cup sour cream
- 8 oz cream cheese

Directions:

Add cream cheese, seasoning, Worcestershire sauce, green onion, and sour cream into the food processor and process until smooth.

Add artichoke into the food processor and process twice.

Transfer mixture into the bowl.

Add shrimp and stir well.

Add shrimp mixture into the slow cooker and cook on low for 40 minutes.

Stir well and serve.

Nutritional Value (Amount per Serving):

Calories 72

Fat 5.3 g

Carbohydrates 2.7 g

Sugar 0.4 g

Protein 4.1 g

Cholesterol 37 mg

46-Spicy Beef Chili

Total Time: 10 hours 10 minutes

Serving Size: 4

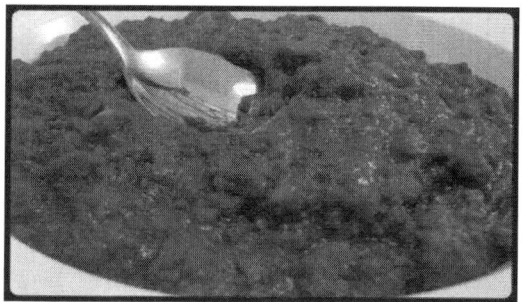

Ingredients:

- 1 lb lean beef, cubed
- 8 oz tomato sauce
- 1/2 Tsp ground chipotle
- 1/2 Tsp cayenne pepper
- 1/2 Tsp white pepper
- 1/2 Tsp black pepper
- 1/2 Tsp oregano
- 1 tbsp paprika
- 2 tbsp chili powder
- 1 tbsp garlic powder
- 2 tbsp onion powder

Directions:

Heat pan over medium high heat.

Place beef on hot pan and brown the beef quickly. Drain the excess grease of beef.

Place brown beef into the slow cooker.

Add remaining ingredients over beef.

Cover slow cooker with lid and cook on low for 10 hours.

Serve and enjoy.

Nutritional Value (Amount per Serving):

Calories 263

Fat 8.2 g

Carbohydrates 11 g

Sugar 4.6 g

Protein 36.7 g

Cholesterol 101 mg

47-Mushrrom Butter Turkey

Total Time: 6 hours 10 minutes

Serving Size: 6

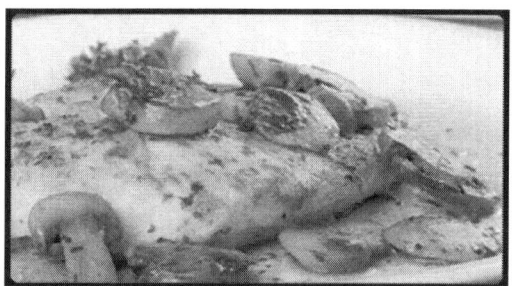

Ingredients:

- 1 1/2 lbs turkey breast cutlets
- 1/4 cup water
- 1/4 Tsp black pepper
- 1 tsp sage, minced
- 8 oz mushrooms, sliced
- 1 medium onion, sliced
- 1 tsp butter
- 1/8 Tsp salt

Directions:

Heat butter in a pan over medium heat.

Add mushrooms and onion in a pan and sauté until softened.

Add half mushroom and onion mixture into the slow cooker.

Add turkey into the slow cooker and sprinkle with pepper, sage, and salt.

Now add remaining mushroom and onion mixture over turkey. Pour water into the slow cooker.

Cover and cook on low for 6 hours.

Serve and enjoy.

Nutritional Value (Amount per Serving):

Calories 142

Fat 1.2 g

Carbohydrates 3.1 g

Sugar 1.4 g

Protein 29.5 g

Cholesterol 47 mg

48-Rosemary Lamb Leg

Total Time: 8 hours 10 minutes

Serving Size: 12

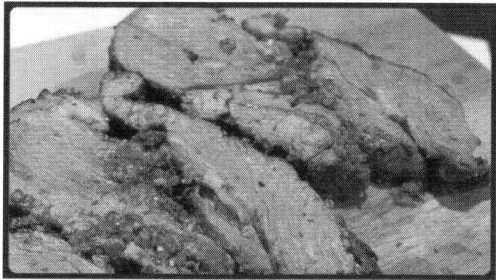

Ingredients:

- 4 lbs lamb leg, boneless and slice of fat
- 1/4 cup water
- 1/4 cup lemon juice
- 1 tbsp rosemary, crushed
- 1 tsp black pepper
- 1/4 Tsp salt

Directions:

Place lamb into the slow cooker.

Add remaining ingredients into the slow cooker over the lamb.

Cover and cook on low for 8 hours.

Remove lamb from slow cooker and sliced.

Serve and enjoy.

Nutritional Value (Amount per Serving):

Calories 275

Fat 10.2 g

Carbohydrates 0.4 g

Sugar 0.1 g

Protein 42.7 g

Cholesterol 132 mg

49-Rosemary Capers Salmon

Total Time: 2 hours 10 minutes

Serving Size: 2

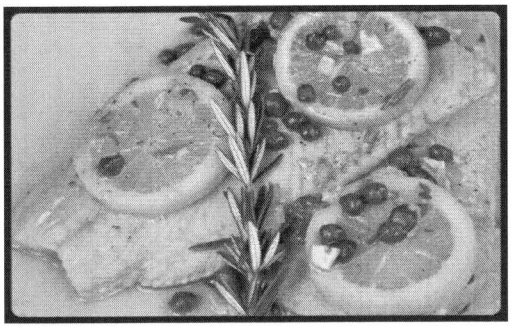

Ingredients:

- 8 oz salmon
- 1/4 Tsp fresh rosemary, minced
- 1 tbsp capers
- 1 fresh lemon, sliced
- 2 tbsp lemon juice
- 1/3 cup water

Directions:

Place salmon into the slow cooker.

Pour lemon juice and water over salmon.

Arrange lemon slices over the top of salmon.

Sprinkle with rosemary and capers.

Cover and cook on low for 2 hours.

Serve and enjoy.

Nutritional Value (Amount per Serving):

Calories 164

Fat 7.3 g

Carbohydrates 3.3 g

Sugar 1.1 g

Protein 22.6 g

Cholesterol 50 mg

50-Onion Sour Cream Zucchini

Total Time: 1 hour 50 minutes

Serving Size: 6

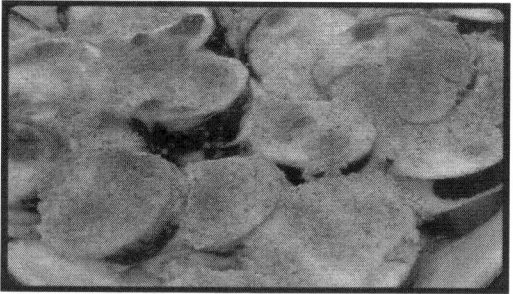

Ingredients:

- 4 cups zucchini, sliced
- 1 cup cheddar cheese, grated
- 1 cup onion, chopped
- 1/4 cup almond milk
- 1 cup sour cream
- 1 tsp salt

Directions:

Microwave zucchini on high for 2 minutes.

Spray slow cooker from inside using cooking spray.

Place zucchini into the slow cooker.

Combine together onion, milk, sour cream, and salt and pour over zucchini.

Cover slow cooker and cook on low for 1 hour.

Sprinkle grated cheese over zucchini and cook for another 30 minutes.

Serve and enjoy.

Nutritional Value (Amount per Serving):

Calories 201

Fat 16.8 g

Carbohydrates 6.7 g

Sugar 2.6 g

Protein 7.3 g

Cholesterol 37 mg

DESSERT RECIPES

51-Yummy Chocolate Cake

Total Time: 3 hours 10 minutes

Serving Size: 10

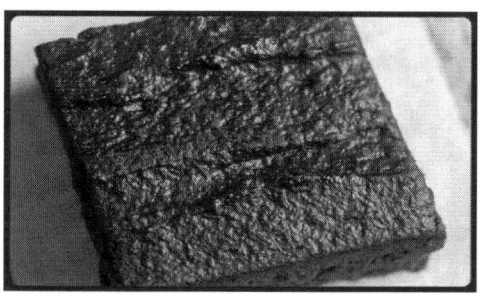

Ingredients:

- 1 cup almond flour
- 1 tsp vanilla extract
- 3/4 cup heavy cream
- 4 eggs
- 1/2 cup butter, melted
- 2 tsp baking powder
- 1/4 cup protein powder
- 2/3 cup cocoa powder, unsweetened
- 3/4 cup Swerve sweetener
- 1/4 Tsp salt

Directions:

Spray slow cooker from inside using cooking spray.

In a mixing bowl, whisk together almond flour, baking powder, protein powder, cocoa powder, sweetener, and salt.

Stir in eggs, vanilla, cream, and butter until well combined.

Pour batter into the slow cooker and cook on low for 3 hours.

Allow to cool for 20 minutes then cut into pieces and serve.

Nutritional Value (Amount per Serving):

Calories 232

Fat 20.8 g

Carbohydrates 6.6 g

Sugar 0.7 g

Protein 9.3 g

Cholesterol 102 mg

52-Cocoa Pudding Cake Delight

Total Time: 3 hours 20 minutes

Serving Size: 6

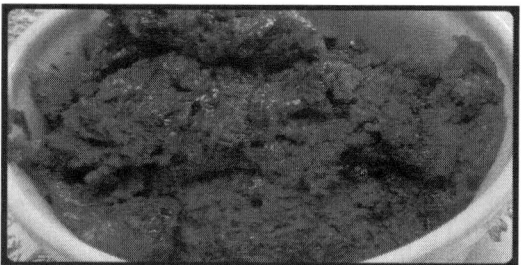

Ingredients:

- 5 eggs
- 1/3 cup almond flour
- 2/3 cup stevia
- 4 tbsp cocoa powder, unsweetened
- 1 tsp vanilla extract
- 2 tbsp instant coffee
- 1/2 cup heavy cream
- 2 oz unsweetened chocolate, chopped
- 3/4 cup butter, cut into pieces
- 1/8 Tsp salt

Directions:

Spray slow cooker form inside using cooking spray.

In a small saucepan, melt chocolate and butter over low heat and set aside to cool.

In a small bowl, whisk together vanilla, coffee, and heavy cream.

In a small bowl, combine almond flour, cocoa, and salt.

Add eggs into the large bowl and beat until creamy then slowly add sweetener and beat again until thickened.

Now slowly add chocolate and butter mixture and stir well.

Stir in almond flour, cocoa, and salt mixture.

Slowly add vanilla, coffee and cream mixture and beat over low speed to well combine.

Pour batter into the slow cooker.

Cook on low for 3 hours.

Cut cake into the pieces and serve.

Nutritional Value (Amount per Serving):

Calories 413

Fat 39 g

Carbohydrates 3.7 g

Sugar 0.8 g

Protein 9 g

Cholesterol 211 mg

53-Gluten Free Lemon Cake

Total Time: 3 hours 10 minutes

Serving Size: 8

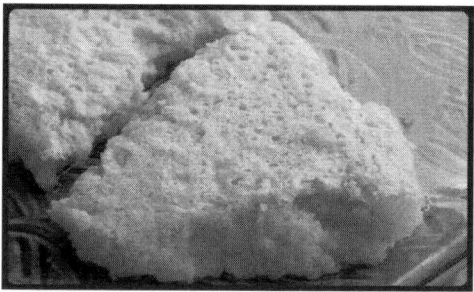

Ingredients:

- 2 eggs
- 1 1/2 cups almond flour
- 2 lemon zest
- 2 tbsp lemon juice
- 1/2 cup whipping cream
- 1/2 cup butter, melted
- 2 tsp baking powder
- 6 tbsp Swerve
- 1/2 cup coconut flour

Directions:

In a medium bowl, combine together almond flour, baking powder, swerve, and coconut flour.

In a large bowl, whisk together eggs, lemon zest, lemon juice, whipping cream, and butter.

Add dry mixture into the wet and fold until well combined.

Pour batter into the slow cooker and cook on high for 3 hours.

Cut into pieces and serve warm.

Nutritional Value (Amount per Serving):

Calories 350

Fat 32 g

Carbohydrates 11 g

Sugar 4.3 g

Protein 7.6 g

Cholesterol 80 mg

54-Yummy Slow Cooker Brownie

Total Time: 4 hours 10 minutes

Serving Size: 10

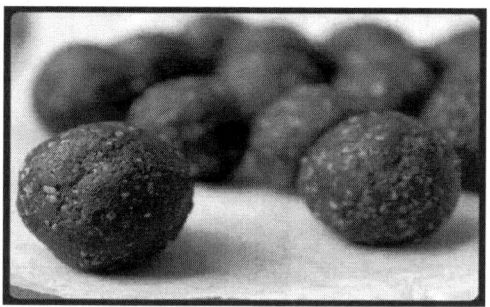

Ingredients:

- 2 eggs
- 1/3 cup water
- 2 tsp vanilla extract
- 1/2 cup coconut oil, melted
- 1/2 cup coconut milk, unsweetened
- 2 tsp baking soda
- 2 tsp baking powder
- 3/4 cup cocoa powder, unsweetened
- 1 cup coconut sugar
- 2 cups almond flour
- 1 tsp salt

Directions:

Grease slow cooker with coconut oil.

Combine together all ingredients and add in the slow cooker.

Cover slow cooker with lid and cook on low for 4 minutes.

Allow cooling mixture for half hour.

Scoop out mixture with large spoon and form into balls.

Serve and enjoy.

Nutritional Value (Amount per Serving):

Calories 289

Fat 26 g

Carbohydrates 11.5 g

Sugar 1.5 g

Protein 7.5 g

Cholesterol 33 mg

55-Moist Blackberry Cake

Total Time: 3 hours 10 minutes

Serving Size: 10

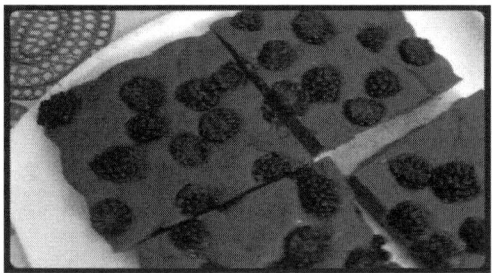

Ingredients:

- 2 cups almond flour
- 1/3 cup sugar-free chocolate chips
- 1 cup blackberries
- 1/2 cup heavy cream
- 1/4 cup butter, melted
- 1/4 cup coconut oil, melted
- 4 eggs
- 2 tsp baking soda
- 1/4 cup protein powder
- 1/2 cup Swerve sweetener
- 1 cup coconut, shredded and unsweetened
- 1/4 Tsp salt

Directions:

Grease slow cooker with melted butter.

Combine together almond flour, baking soda, protein powder, sweetener, coconut, and salt.

Stir in heavy cream, butter, coconut oil, and eggs until combined.

Add chocolate chips and blackberries and fold well.

Pour batter into the slow cooker and cook on low for 3 hours.

Allow cooling completely then cut into the pieces.

Serve and enjoy.

Nutritional Value (Amount per Serving):

Calories 385

Fat 30 g

Carbohydrates 11 g

Sugar 5 g

Protein 21.4 g

Cholesterol 87 mg

SOUP RECIPES

56-Ground Beef Zucchini Soup

Total Time: 5 hours 10 minutes

Serving Size: 5

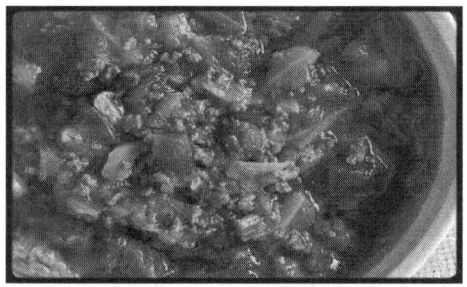

Ingredients:

- 1 lb ground beef
- 1/2 Tsp basil, dried
- 1/2 Tsp oregano, dried
- 1 tbsp garlic, minced
- 28 oz tomatoes, diced
- 1/2 cup vegetable broth
- 1 celery stalk, diced
- 1 carrot, diced
- 1 onion, diced
- 2 small zucchini, diced

Directions:

Heat pan over medium high heat.

Brown ground beef in hot pan.

Add 3 cups water into the saucepan and bring to boil.

Add ground beef in boiling water and pour into the slow cooker.

Add remaining ingredients into the slow cooker and stir well.

Cover and cook on low for 5 hours.

Stir well and serve.

Nutritional Value (Amount per Serving):

Calories 226

Fat 6.3 g

Carbohydrates 11.9 g

Sugar 6.7 g

Protein 30.5 g

Cholesterol 81 mg

57-Yummy Chicken Vegetable Soup

Total Time: 6 hours 10 minutes

Serving Size: 6

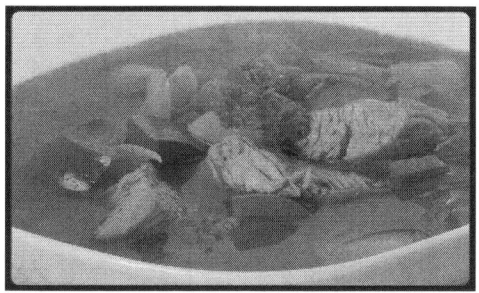

Ingredients:

- 4 cups chicken, boneless, cooked and diced
- 2 tbsp lime juice
- 1/2 cup fresh cilantro, chopped
- 1 tsp chili powder
- 1 tbsp cumin
- 1 3/4 cups tomato juice
- 1/4 cup jalapeno, diced
- 1/2 cup tomato, diced
- 4 tsp garlic, minced
- 2/3 cups onion, diced
- 1 1/2 cups carrot, diced
- 6 cups chicken stock
- 2 tsp sea salt

Directions:

Add all ingredients into the slow cooker and stir well.

Cover and cook on low for 6 hours.

Stir well and serve.

Nutritional Value (Amount per Serving):

Calories 192

Fat 3.8 g

Carbohydrates 9.8 g

Sugar 5.7 g

Protein 29.2 g

Cholesterol 72 mg

58-Kale Turkey Soup

Total Time: 8 hours 10 minutes

Serving Size: 6

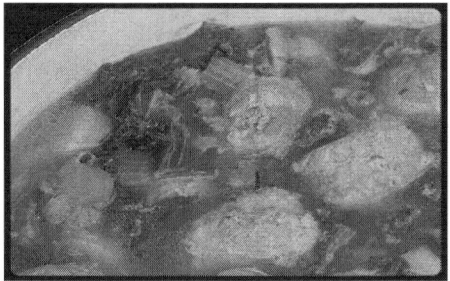

Ingredients:

- 3 cups turkey meat, cut into pieces

- 3 cups kale, chopped

- 2 rosemary sprigs

- 4 cups chicken stock

- 2 garlic cloves, minced

- 2 carrots, peeled and sliced

- 1/2 onion, chopped

- 1/2 tbsp olive oil

Directions:

Heat olive oil in the pan over medium heat.

Add onion to the pan and sauté until softened.

Add carrots and garlic and sauté for 2 minutes.

Add onion mixture into the slow cooker then add all remaining ingredients and stir well.

Cover slow cooker with lid and cook on low for 8 hours.

Discard rosemary and serve.

Nutritional Value (Amount per Serving):

Calories 166

Fat 5.1 g

Carbohydrates 7.2 g

Sugar 1.9 g

Protein 22.3 g

Cholesterol 53 mg

59-Creamy Tomato Basil Soup

Total Time: 4 hours 10 minutes

Serving Size: 6

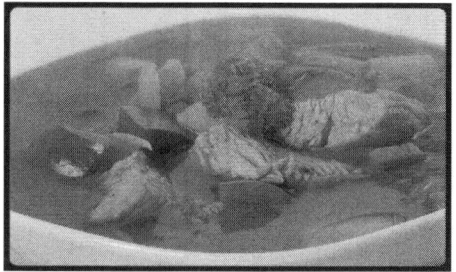

Ingredients:

- 28 oz tomatoes, diced
- 1/2 cup parmesan cheese, grated
- 1/2 cup heavy cream
- 1/4 Tsp red pepper flakes
- 1 tbsp onion powder
- 1/2 tbsp thyme, dried
- 10 basil leaves
- 3 tbsp garlic, chopped
- 28 oz whole tomatoes, diced

Directions:

Add all ingredients except heavy cream and cheese into the slow cooker and stir well.

Use a blender to blend.

Cover and cook on low for 4 hours.

Stir in cheese and heavy cream.

Serve and enjoy.

Nutritional Value (Amount per Serving):

Calories 117

Fat 5.9 g

Carbohydrates 13 g

Sugar 7.4 g

Protein 5.7 g

Cholesterol 19 mg

60-Creamy Coconut Tomato Curried Soup

Total Time: 4 hours 10 minutes

Serving Size: 8

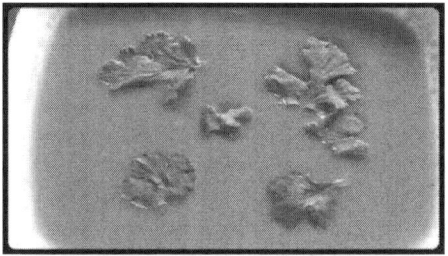

Ingredients:

- 4 lbs tomatoes, cored and diced
- 2 tbsp onion, minced
- 1 tsp garlic, minced
- 2 tsp curry powder
- 2 cups coconut milk
- 1 cup water
- 1 tsp salt

Directions:

Add all ingredients into the slow cooker and stir well.

Cover and cook on high for 4 hours.

Using blender puree the soup until smooth.

Stir well and serve.

Nutritional Value (Amount per Serving):

Calories 182

Fat 14.8 g

Carbohydrates 12 g

Sugar 8.1 g

Protein 3.5 g

Cholesterol 0 mg

61-Creamy Cauliflower Curried Soup

Total Time: 8 hours 10 minutes

Serving Size: 4

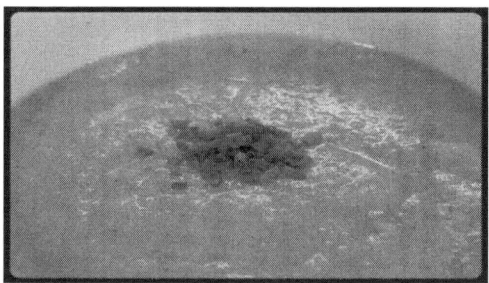

Ingredients:

- 1 lb cauliflower, cut into florets
- 1/4 Tsp cumin
- 3 tsp curry powder
- 2 garlic cloves, minced
- 1 onion, minced
- 2 1/2 cups water

Directions:

Add all ingredients into the slow cooker and stir well.

Cover and cook on low for 8 hours.

Using blender puree the soup until smooth.

Stir well and serve.

Nutritional Value (Amount per Serving):

Calories 47

Fat 0.4 g

Carbohydrates 10 g

Sugar 4 g

Protein 2.9 g

Cholesterol 0 mg

62-Creamy Mushrooms Soup

Total Time: 8 hours 10 minutes

Serving Size: 6

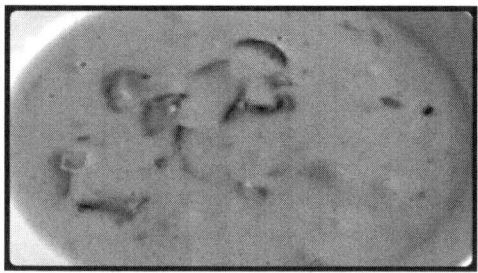

Ingredients:

- 2 oz dried mushrooms, soaked in water about 10 minutes
- 1/2 cup heavy cream
- 4 fresh thyme sprigs
- 4 garlic cloves, crushed
- 1 onion, diced
- 1 tbsp butter
- 4 cups vegetable broth
- 4 cups mushrooms, sliced
- Pepper
- Salt

Directions:

Add mushrooms, thyme, garlic, onion, butter, and broth into the slow cooker and stir well.

Season with pepper and salt.

Cover slow cooker and cook on low for 8 hours.

Remove thyme sprigs from slow cooker.

Add 2 cups of soup mixture into the blender and blend until smooth.

Return blended mixture to the slow cooker.

Stir in heavy cream

Serve warm and enjoy.

Nutritional Value (Amount per Serving):

Calories 110

Fat 7 g

Carbohydrates 5 g

Sugar 2 g

Protein 6 g

Cholesterol 19 mg

63-Garlic Butter Sauerkraut Soup

Total Time: 8 hours 10 minutes

Serving Size: 12

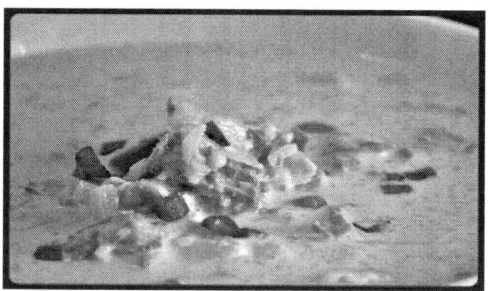

Ingredients:

- 1 lb sauerkraut
- 8 oz Swiss cheese, shredded
- 2 cups heavy cream
- 1 tbsp mustard seeds
- 1 tsp dill seeds
- 1 tsp coriander seeds
- 1/2 Tsp celery seeds
- 2 lbs corned beef, diced
- 2 tbsp butter
- 3 garlic cloves, minced
- 1 medium onion, diced
- 8 cups beef broth

Directions:

Melt 1 tbsp butter in a pan over medium heat.

Add onion in a pan and cook until translucent.

Add garlic and sauté for a minute.

Add broth, corned beef, onion garlic mixture, seeds, sauerkraut, and remaining butter into the slow cooker. Stir well.

Cover and cook on low for 7 hours.

One hour before serving add cheese and cream.

Stir well and serve.

Nutritional Value (Amount per Serving):

Calories 328

Fat 25.3 g

Carbohydrates 5 g

Sugar 2.5 g

Protein 19.3 g

Cholesterol 97 mg

64-Creamy Asparagus Soup

Total Time: 4 hours 10 minutes

Serving Size: 4

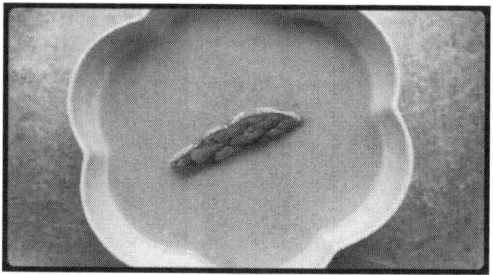

Ingredients:

- 1 lb asparagus, trimmed and chopped
- 2 tbsp butter
- 1/2 cup onion, chopped
- 2 cups chicken broth
- 1/4 Tsp pepper
- 1/2 Tsp salt

Directions:

Add all ingredients into the slow cooker and stir well.

Cover and cook on high for 4 hours.

Using blender puree the soup until smooth.

Stir well and serve.

Nutritional Value (Amount per Serving):

Calories 99

Fat 6.6 g

Carbohydrates 6.3 g

Sugar 3.1 g

Protein 5.1 g

Cholesterol 15 mg

65-4 Ingredients Chicken Soup

Total Time: 4 hours 10 minutes

Serving Size: 6

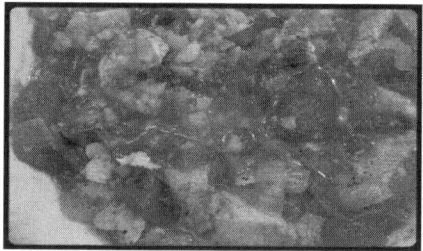

Ingredients:

- 1 1/2 lbs chicken, skinless and boneless, cut into pieces
- 8 oz pepper jack cheese, shredded
- 15 oz chicken broth
- 15 oz chunky salsa

Directions:

Place chicken into the slow cooker then pours remaining ingredients over the chicken.

Cover and cook on high for 4 hours.

Using fork shred the chicken and stirs well.

Serve and enjoy.

Nutritional Value (Amount per Serving):

Calories 400

Fat 22.8 g

Carbohydrates 7.4 g

Sugar 4.7 g

Protein 38 g

Cholesterol 137 mg

66-Bacon Chicken Leek Soup

Total Time: 1 hour 20 minutes

Serving Size: 4

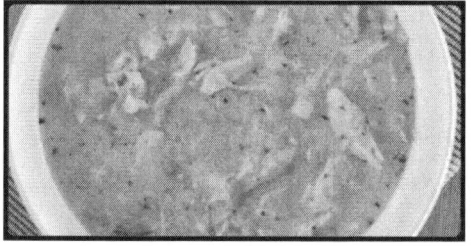

Ingredients:

- 2 cups chicken, cooked
- 1 tbsp fish sauce
- 1 cup coconut milk
- 6 cups chicken broth
- 2 tsp mix herbs
- 1 tsp mustard
- 1 garlic clove, crushed
- 3 bacon pieces, chopped
- 2 leeks, sliced
- 1 onion, chopped
- Pepper
- Salt

Directions:

Spray slow cooker from inside using cooking spray and set on high.

Add onion and bacon and cook until lightly golden.

Add garlic and leek and cook until softened.

Add mustard, herbs, fish sauce, broth, and mix herbs into the slow cooker and stir well.

Cover slow cooker with lid and cook on high for 1 hour.

Add coconut milk and chicken into the slow cooker and stir well.

Season with pepper salt.

Serve and enjoy.

Nutritional Value (Amount per Serving):

Calories 219

Fat 10 g

Carbohydrates 12 g

Sugar 2.2 g

Protein 19 g

Cholesterol 64 mg

67-Spinach Chicken Soup

Total Time: 4 hours 10 minutes

Serving Size: 6

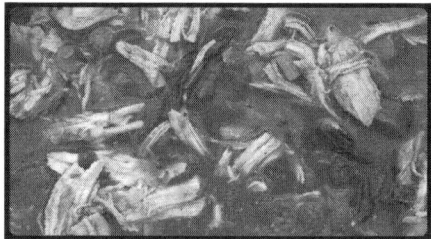

Ingredients:

- 4 chicken breasts
- 4 cups chicken broth
- 28 oz tomatoes, crushed
- 1 1/2 tbsp herb de Provence
- 1 bay leaf
- 1/4 cup fresh spinach
- 4 celery stalks, chopped
- 1/2 onion, chopped
- 6 carrots, chopped
- 1/2 Tsp black pepper
- 1 tsp salt

Directions:

Add all ingredients except spinach into the slow cooker and stir well.

Cover and cook on high for 4 hours.

Remove chicken from slow cooker and shred using a fork.

Return shredded chicken to the slow cooker with spinach and stir well.

Serve and enjoy.

Nutritional Value (Amount per Serving):

Calories 227

Fat 6.8 g

Carbohydrates 13 g

Sugar 7 g

Protein 27 g

Cholesterol 67 mg

68-Zucchini Turkey Soup

Total Time: 3 hours 30 minutes

Serving Size: 8

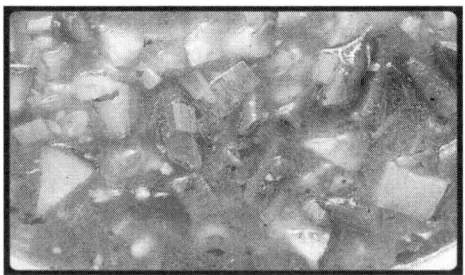

Ingredients:

- 2 cups zucchini, sliced
- 2 cups turkey, cooked and chopped
- 4 cups water
- 1 tsp Worcestershire sauce
- 1 tbsp chicken bouillon granules
- 1/2 cup onions, chopped
- 8 oz tomato sauce
- 8 oz frozen green beans
- 3 oz cream cheese, softened
- 1/8 Tsp black pepper
- 1/4 Tsp salt

Directions:

Add all ingredients except cream cheese into the slow cooker and stir well.

Cover and cook on high for 3 hours.

Blend 1 cup soup with cream cheese and return to the slow cooker.

Stir well and cook for another 20 minutes.

Serve warm and enjoy.

Nutritional Value (Amount per Serving):

Calories 120

Fat 5.6 g

Carbohydrates 5.6 g

Sugar 2.6 g

Protein 12.4 g

Cholesterol 38 mg

69-Vegetable Pork Soup

Total Time: 6 hours 20 minutes

Serving Size: 6

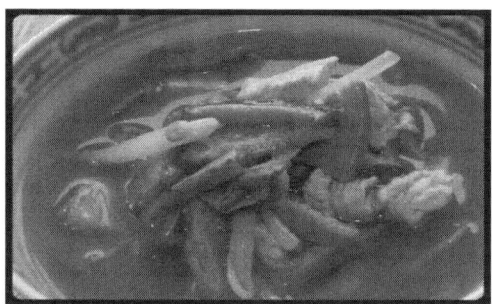

Ingredients:

- 1 lb lean pork, cut into cubes
- 1 cup bean sprouts
- 1 cup mushrooms, sliced
- 10 oz beef broth
- 1/2 Tsp ginger root, chopped
- 3 tbsp soy sauce
- 1 garlic clove, chopped
- 4 green onions, chopped
- 2 medium carrots cut into strips
- 1/8 Tsp black pepper

Directions:

Heat pan over medium heat.

Add meat to hot pan and cook for 10 minutes.

Add meat and remaining ingredients except bean sprouts and mushrooms into the slow cooker. Stir well.

Cover and cook on low for 5 hours.

Stir in bean sprouts and sliced mushrooms.

Cover and cook on low for another 1 hour.

Stir well and serve.

Nutritional Value (Amount per Serving):

Calories 194

Fat 7.9 g

Carbohydrates 5.4 g

Sugar 1.7 g

Protein 25.1 g

Cholesterol 60 mg

70-Creamy Avocado Soup

Total Time: 8 hours 10 minutes

Serving Size: 8

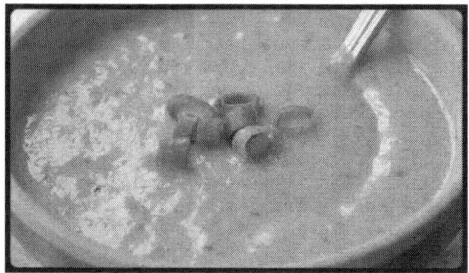

Ingredients:

- 3 ripe avocados, smashed
- 1 tbsp fresh lime juice
- 1 bay leaf
- 1 tsp oregano
- 1 tbsp ground cumin
- 3 garlic cloves, minced
- 1 large onion, chopped
- 32 oz chicken stock
- Pepper
- Salt

Directions:

Add all ingredients into the slow cooker and stir well.

Cover and cook on low for 8 hours.

Discard bay leaf and using blender puree the soup until smooth.

Serve warm and enjoy.

Nutritional Value (Amount per Serving):

Calories 171

Fat 15.2 g

Carbohydrates 9.4 g

Sugar 1.6 g

Protein 2.2 g

Cholesterol 0 mg

71-Healthy Green Bean Tomato Soup

Total Time: 6 hours 10 minutes

Serving Size: 8

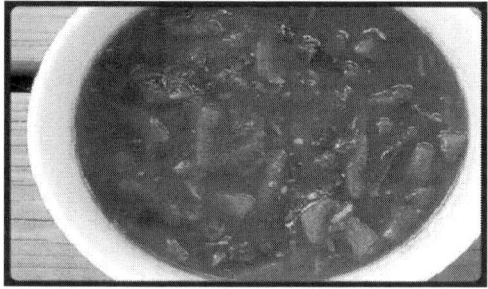

Ingredients:

- 3 cups fresh tomatoes, diced
- 1 lb fresh green beans, cut into 1-inch pieces
- 1 tsp basil, dried
- 1 garlic clove, minced
- 6 cups chicken broth
- 1 cup carrots, chopped
- 1 cup onions, chopped
- 1/4 Tsp black pepper
- 1/2 Tsp salt

Directions:

Add all ingredients into the slow cooker and stir well.

Cover slow cooker with lid and cook on low for 6 hours.

Stir well and serve.

Nutritional Value (Amount per Serving):

Calories 71

Fat 1.3 g

Carbohydrates 10.2 g

Sugar 4.4 g

Protein 5.6 g

Cholesterol 0 mg

72-Ginger Carrot Soup

Total Time: 3 hours 10 minutes

Serving Size: 4

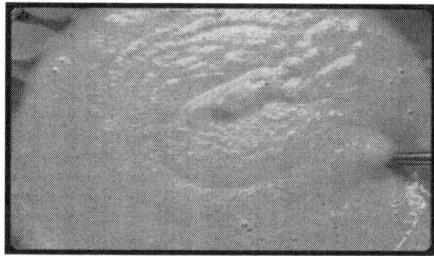

Ingredients:

- 6 carrots, chopped
- 1 tsp paprika
- 1 garlic clove
- 1/3 cup water
- 1 tbsp ginger, chopped
- 1 cup coconut milk
- 1 tsp salt

Directions:

Add all ingredients into the slow cooker and stir well.

Cover and cook on low for 4 hours.

Using blender puree the soup until smooth.

Serve warm and enjoy.

Nutritional Value (Amount per Serving):

Calories 183

Fat 14.5 g

Carbohydrates 13 g

Sugar 6.6 g

Protein 2.4 g

Cholesterol 0 mg

73-Lemon Garlic Lamb Stew

Total Time: 8 hours 10 minutes

Serving Size: 2

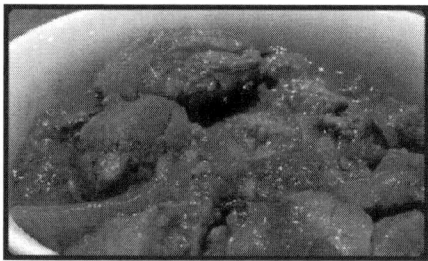

Ingredients:

- 1/2 lb lean lamb, boneless and cubed
- 2 fresh thyme sprigs
- 1/4 Tsp turmeric
- 1/4 cup green olives, sliced
- 2 tbsp lemon juice
- 1/2 onion, chopped
- 2 garlic cloves, minced
- 1/2 Tsp black pepper
- 1/4 Tsp salt

Directions:

Add all ingredients into the slow cooker and stir well.

Cover slow cooker with lid and cook on low for 8 hours.

Stir well and serve.

Nutritional Value (Amount per Serving):

Calories 297

Fat 20.3 g

Carbohydrates 5.4 g

Sugar 1.5 g

Protein 21 g

Cholesterol 80 mg

74-Herb Mushroom Chicken Stew

Total Time: 4 hours 10 minutes

Serving Size: 6

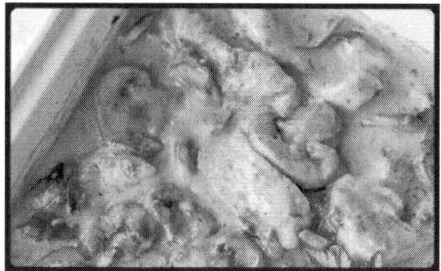

Ingredients:

- 1 1/2 lbs chicken breasts, skinless and boneless, cut into pieces
- 1 tsp basil, dried
- 1 tsp marjoram, dried
- 1 tsp oregano, dried
- 1 tsp thyme, dried
- 3/4 cup water
- 6 oz tomato paste
- 4 garlic cloves, diced
- 1 cup bell pepper, diced
- 3 cups zucchini, diced
- 1 medium onion, diced
- 8 oz mushrooms, sliced

- 2 tbsp olive oil
- 2 tsp salt

Directions:

Heat 1 tbsp olive oil in a pan over medium heat.

Add chicken to the pan and cook until brown then transfer to slow cooker.

In the same pan, sauté garlic, green pepper, zucchini, onions, and mushrooms with remaining olive oil.

Transfer pan mixture into the slow cooker.

Add water, seasoning, tomato paste, and tomatoes into the slow cooker.

Cover slow cooker with lid and cook on low for 4 hours.

Stir well and serve.

Nutritional Value (Amount per Serving):

Calories 314

Fat 13.5 g

Carbohydrates 12 g

Sugar 6.9 g

Protein 36.5 g

Cholesterol 101 mg

75-Tomato Thyme Lamb Stew

Total Time: 6 hours 10 minutes

Serving Size: 6

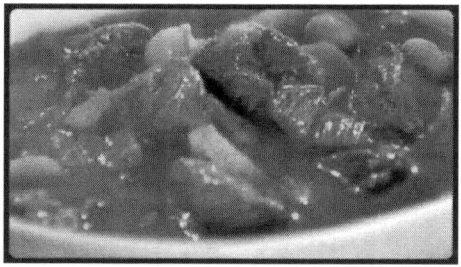

Ingredients:

- 3 lbs lamb shoulder, cut into pieces
- 1 bay leaf
- 1/2 Tsp thyme, dried
- 1 tsp fresh thyme
- 1 tsp oregano, dried
- 2 onions, diced
- 6 garlic cloves, chopped
- 28 oz tomatoes, diced
- 2 cups white wine
- 4 cups beef broth
- Pepper
- Salt

Directions:

Add all ingredients into the slow cooker and stir well.

Cover slow cooker with lid and cook on low for 6 hours.

Discard bay leaf.

Stir well and serve.

Nutritional Value (Amount per Serving):

Calories 557

Fat 17.9 g

Carbohydrates 12 g

Sugar 6.2 g

Protein 68.8 g

Cholesterol 204 mg

CHICKEN RECIPES

76-Tasty Jerk Chicken Wings

Total Time: 5 hours 10 minutes

Serving Size: 4

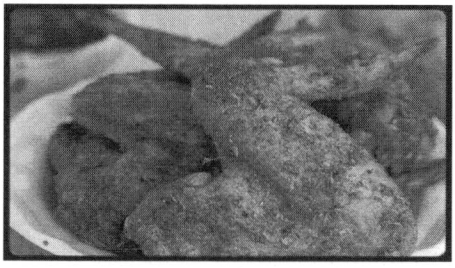

Ingredients:

- 20 oz chicken breasts
- 2 tsp garlic powder
- 2 tsp white pepper
- 2 tsp thyme
- 2 tsp onion powder
- 1 tsp cayenne pepper
- 4 tsp paprika
- 1 tsp black pepper
- 2 tsp salt

Directions:

In a small bowl, combine together all spices and rub over chicken.

Place chicken into the slow cooker.

Cover slow cooker with lid and cook on low for 5 hours.

Serve and enjoy.

Nutritional Value (Amount per Serving):

Calories 291

Fat 11 g

Carbohydrates 4.8 g

Sugar 1.1 g

Protein 42 g

Cholesterol 126 mg

77-Creamy Chicken Curry

Total Time: 4 hours 10 minutes

Serving Size: 6

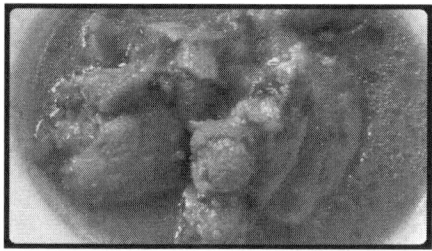

Ingredients:

- 3 lbs chicken thighs, skinless and boneless
- 3 tbsp green curry paste
- 2 cups coconut milk

Directions:

Add all ingredients into the slow cooker and stir well.

Cover slow cooker with lid and cook on low for 4 hours.

Using fork shred the chicken.

Stir well and serve.

Nutritional Value (Amount per Serving):

Calories 637

Fat 37.4 g

Carbohydrates 6.7 g

Sugar 2.7 g

Protein 67.4 g

Cholesterol 202 mg

78-Yummy Chicken Fajita

Total Time: 6 hours 10 minutes

Serving Size: 6

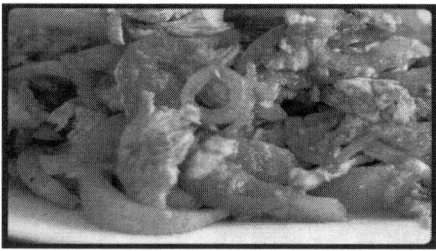

Ingredients:

- 2 lbs chicken, skinless and boneless
- 14 oz tomatoes, diced
- 1/2 Tsp chipotle chili powder
- 1/2 Tsp cumin
- 1 tsp oregano, dried
- 1 tsp ground coriander
- 2 cups bell peppers, sliced
- 4 garlic cloves, minced
- 1 small onion, sliced
- 1 tsp kosher salt

Directions:

Place chicken into the slow cooker then tops with remaining ingredients.

Cover slow cooker with lid and cook on low for 6 hours.

Stir well and serve.

Nutritional Value (Amount per Serving):

Calories 262

Fat 4.9 g

Carbohydrates 7.6 g

Sugar 4.3 g

Protein 45.1 g

Cholesterol 116 mg

79-Lemon Garlic Chicken

Total Time: 5 hours 10 minutes

Serving Size: 6

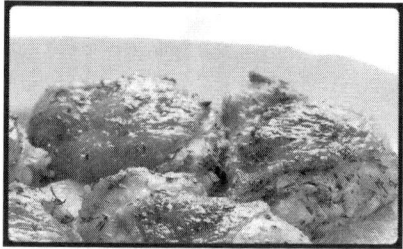

Ingredients:

- 2 lbs chicken breasts, skinless, boneless and halves
- 1 tbsp fresh parsley, minced
- 1 tsp chicken bouillon granules
- 3 tbsp fresh lemon juice
- 1/4 cup water
- 2 tbsp butter
- 1 tsp oregano, dried
- 1/4 Tsp black pepper
- 1/2 Tsp salt

Directions:

In a small bowl, combine together oregano, black pepper, and salt and rub over chicken.

Heat butter in a pan over medium heat.

Add chicken in pan and cook until brown.

Transfer chicken into the slow cooker.

Add lemon juice, water, and granules in the pan and bring to boil over high heat.

Pour lemon mixture over the chicken.

Cover and cook on low for 5 hours.

Garnish with parsley and serve.

Nutritional Value (Amount per Serving):

Calories 324

Fat 15.1 g

Carbohydrates 0.4 g

Sugar 0.2 g

Protein 43.9 g

Cholesterol 145 mg

80-Easy Thai Chicken Curry

Total Time: 2 hours 10 minutes

Serving Size: 4

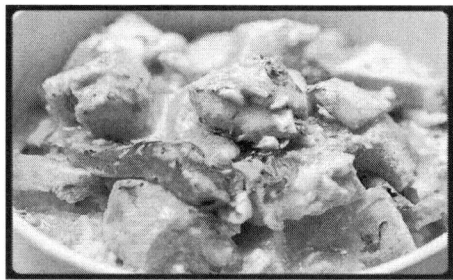

Ingredients:

- 1 lb chicken thighs, skinless and boneless
- 2 garlic cloves, minced
- 1 tbsp fish sauce
- 1 tbsp coconut amino
- 1 tbsp curry paste
- 1/2 cup chicken stock
- 14 oz coconut milk
- Pepper
- Salt

Directions:

Add all ingredients into the slow cooker and stir well.

Cover slow cooker with lid and cook on high for 2 hours.

Stir well and serve.

Nutritional Value (Amount per Serving):

Calories 478

Fat 34.3 g

Carbohydrates 8.1 g

Sugar 3.6 g

Protein 35.7 g

Cholesterol 101 mg

81-Simple Tarragon Chicken

Total Time: 8 hours 10 minutes

Serving Size: 4

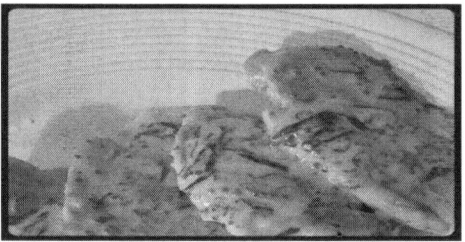

Ingredients:

- 8 oz chicken breasts
- 1 medium onion, sliced
- 2 cups fresh tarragon
- 1/4 Tsp black pepper
- 1/4 Tsp salt

Directions:

Place chicken into the slow cooker.

Top chicken with remaining ingredients.

Cover slow cooker with lid and cook on low for 8 hours.

Remove chicken skin and discard onions and tarragon.

Serve and enjoy.

Nutritional Value (Amount per Serving):

Calories 162

Fat 5.3 g

Carbohydrates 9.9 g

Sugar 1.2 g

Protein 20 g

Cholesterol 50 mg

82-Tasty Herb Shallot Chicken

Total Time: 4 hours 10 minutes

Serving Size: 4

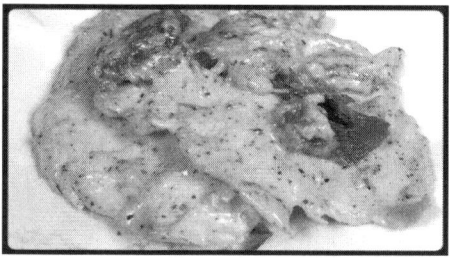

Ingredients:

- 1 lb chicken breast tenderloins, skinless and boneless
- 1 cup chicken stock
- 1 tbsp fresh rosemary, minced
- 1 tbsp fresh lemon juice
- 2 tbsp white wine vinegar
- 1 shallot, minced
- 4 garlic cloves, minced

Directions:

Add all ingredients into the slow cooker and stir well.

Cover and cook on low for 4 hours.

Stir well and serve.

Nutritional Value (Amount per Serving):

Calories 122

Fat 0.8 g

Carbohydrates 4 g

Sugar 0.3 g

Protein 23 g

Cholesterol 71 mg

83-Spinach Garlic Chicken

Total Time: 6 hours 25 minutes

Serving Size: 4

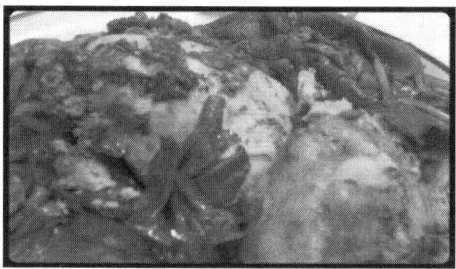

Ingredients:

- 3/4 lb chicken breasts, skinless, boneless and cut into strips
- 5 oz baby spinach
- 1 tbsp fresh parsley, minced
- 1 tbsp fresh oregano, minced
- 4 garlic cloves, minced
- 1/4 cup balsamic vinegar
- 1/2 Tsp black pepper

Directions:

Add all ingredients except spinach into the slow cooker and stir well.

Cover and cook on low for 6 hours.

Stir in spinach and cook for another 15 minutes.

Stir well and serve.

Nutritional Value (Amount per Serving):

Calories 182

Fat 6.6 g

Carbohydrates 3.4 g

Sugar 0.3 g

Protein 26 g

Cholesterol 76 mg

84-Celery Carrot Whole Chicken

Total Time: 8 hours 5 minutes

Serving Size: 8

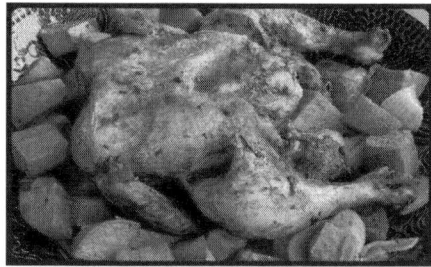

Ingredients:

- 4 lbs whole chicken
- 1 cup water
- 1 medium onion, quartered
- 1 celery stalk
- 1 medium carrot, sliced

Directions:

Place chicken into the slow cooker.

Place vegetables around the chicken.

Pour water into the slow cooker.

Cover and cook on low for 8 hours.

Remove chicken skin and serve.

Nutritional Value (Amount per Serving):

Calories 440

Fat 16.8 g

Carbohydrates 2.1 g

Sugar 1 g

Protein 65.8 g

Cholesterol 202 mg

85-Cinnamon Coconut Chicken Curry

Total Time: 6 hours 10 minutes

Serving Size: 6

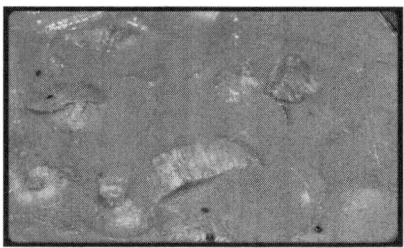

Ingredients:

- 3 lbs chicken thighs, skinless, boneless and cubed
- 1 1/2 cups water
- 2 tbsp red pepper flakes
- 1 tsp mustard seeds
- 1 tsp cumin seeds
- 1/2 Tsp ground cloves
- 1/4 Tsp nutmeg
- 1 tsp cinnamon
- 2 cups shredded coconut, toasted
- 1 tbsp fresh ginger, minced
- 4 garlic cloves, minced
- 2 medium onions, diced
- 1 tsp olive oil

- 1/2 Tsp salt

Directions:

Heat olive oil in a pan over medium heat.

Add onion and garlic to the pan and sauté for 3 minutes.

Add onion and garlic mixture into the slow cooker with remaining ingredients and stir well.

Cover slow cooker and cook on low for 6 hours.

Stir well and serve.

Nutritional Value (Amount per Serving):

Calories 339

Fat 16.3 g

Carbohydrates 6.4 g

Sugar 2.1 g

Protein 40.6 g

Cholesterol 121 mg

86-Delicious Roasted Turkey Breast

Total Time: 8 hours 10 minutes

Serving Size: 10

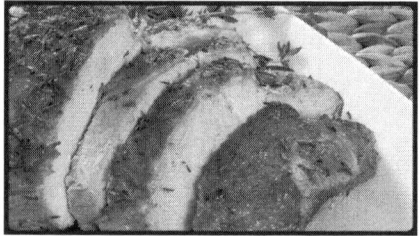

Ingredients:

- 6 lbs turkey breasts
- 1/2 tbsp mustard seeds
- 1/2 tbsp celery flakes
- 1/2 tbsp parsley, dried
- 1/2 cup fresh thyme, minced
- 2 onions, sliced
- 1/2 tbsp black pepper
- 1/2 tbsp salt

Directions:

Arrange onion slices on the bottom of slow cooker.

Make a slit in turkey skin and spread thyme in the skin.

In a small bowl, combine together mustard seeds, celery flakes, parsley, pepper, and salt and rub all over turkey.

Place turkey into the slow cooker.

Cover and cook on low for 8 hours.

Serve and enjoy.

Nutritional Value (Amount per Serving):

Calories 482

Fat 14 g

Carbohydrates 4 g

Sugar 1 g

Protein 80.4 g

Cholesterol 206 mg

87-Celery Garlic Chicken

Total Time: 6 hours 10 minutes

Serving Size: 6

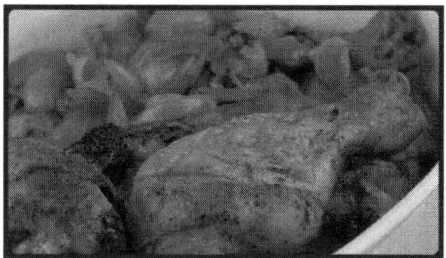

Ingredients:

- 6 chicken breasts, skinless, boneless and halves
- 1 lemon juice
- 4 celery ribs, chopped
- 20 garlic cloves
- 1 tsp oregano, dried
- 2 tsp basil leaves, dried
- 2 tbsp dried parsley, chopped
- 1/4 cup dry white wine
- 1/8 Tsp red pepper flakes

Directions:

In a large bowl, combine together wine, red pepper flakes, oregano, basil, and parsley.

Add celery and garlic cloves into the slow cooker and stir well.

Place chicken into the bowl mixture and coat well.

Add chicken into the slow cooker and sprinkle lemon juice over the chicken.

Cover slow cooker and cook on low for 6 hours.

Serve and enjoy.

Nutritional Value (Amount per Serving):

Calories 246

Fat 8.6 g

Carbohydrates 4.8 g

Sugar 0.7 g

Protein 33.8 g

Cholesterol 101 mg

88-Easy Lemon Chicken

Total Time: 4 hours 10 minutes

Serving Size: 6

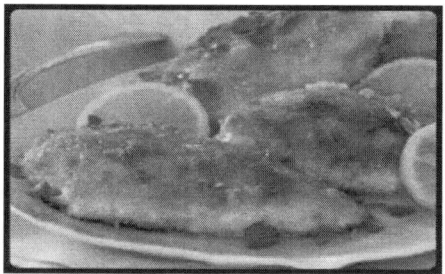

Ingredients:

- 6 chicken breasts, skinless, boneless and halves
- 2 tsp fresh parsley, minced
- 2 tsp chicken bouillon granules
- 2 garlic cloves, minced
- 3 tbsp fresh lemon juice
- 1/4 cup water
- 1 tsp oregano, dried
- 1/4 Tsp black pepper
- 1/2 Tsp salt

Directions:

Combine together oregano, pepper, and salt and rub over chicken.

Heat pan over medium heat. Place chicken on pan and cook until brown.

Place chicken into the slow cooker.

Combine together water, bouillon, garlic, and lemon juice and pour over chicken.

Cover slow cooker and cook on low for 4 hours.

Add parsley and stir well.

Serve and enjoy.

Nutritional Value (Amount per Serving):

Calories 220

Fat 8.5 g

Carbohydrates 0.8 g

Sugar 0.2 g

Protein 33 g

Cholesterol 101 mg

89-Creamy Lemon Dill Chicken

Total Time: 4 hours 10 minutes

Serving Size: 4

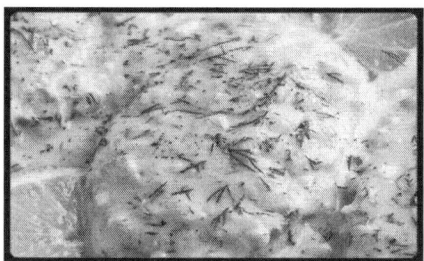

Ingredients:

- 16 oz chicken breasts, skinless, boneless and halves
- 1 tsp lemon zest
- 1 tsp lemon pepper seasoning
- 1 tbsp fresh dill, minced
- 1 cup sour cream

Directions:

In a bowl, combine together lemon zest, lemon pepper seasoning, dill, and sour cream.

Pour half bowl mixture into the slow cooker.

Place chicken into the slow cooker then pours remaining bowl mixture over the chicken.

Cover slow cooker and cook on low for 4 hours.

Serve and enjoy.

Nutritional Value (Amount per Serving):

Calories 342

Fat 20.5 g

Carbohydrates 3.3 g

Sugar 0.1 g

Protein 34.9 g

Cholesterol 126 mg

90-3 Ingredients Italian Chicken

Total Time: 6 hours 5 minutes

Serving Size: 4

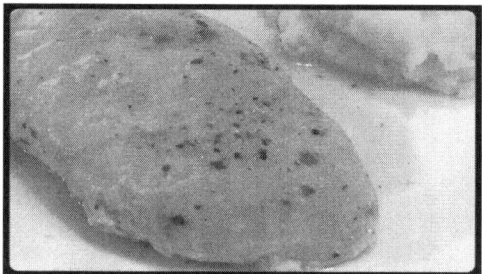

Ingredients:

- 16 oz chicken breasts, skinless, boneless, and halves
- 1 cup chicken stock
- 1 package Italian dressing mix

Directions:

Place chicken into the slow cooker.

Sprinkle dressing mix over the chicken.

Pour chicken stock into the slow cooker.

Cover slow cooker and cook on low for 6 hours.

Serve and enjoy.

Nutritional Value (Amount per Serving):

Calories 249

Fat 8.9 g

Carbohydrates 6.8 g

Sugar 0.2 g

Protein 33.3 g

Cholesterol 101 mg

91-Oregano Cheese Chicken

Total Time: 4 hours 10 minutes

Serving Size: 8

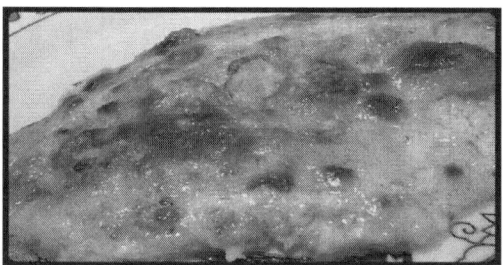

Ingredients:

- 2 lbs chicken breasts, skinless, boneless and halves
- 1/4 Tsp paprika
- 2 tsp oregano, dried
- 1/2 cup parmesan cheese, grated
- 1 cup mayonnaise
- 1/2 cup water
- 1/4 Tsp black pepper

Directions:

Place chicken into the slow cooker.

Pour water into the slow cooker.

Cover slow cooker and cook on high for 2 hours.

Combine remaining ingredients and spread over the chicken.

Cover again and cook on high for 2 hours.

Serve and enjoy.

Nutritional Value (Amount per Serving):

Calories 392

Fat 22.3 g

Carbohydrates 8.4 g

Sugar 1.9 g

Protein 39.1 g

Cholesterol 124 mg

92-Healthy Vegetable Chicken

Total Time: 4 hours 10 minutes

Serving Size: 6

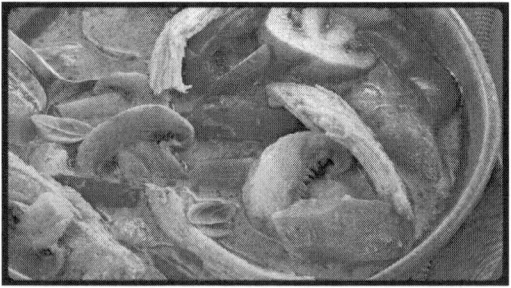

Ingredients:

- 24 oz chicken breasts, skinless, boneless and halves
- 2 tsp dried parsley
- 1/2 Tsp dried basil
- 1/2 cup white wine
- 1 cup water
- 1/4 Tsp red pepper flakes
- 2 celery ribs, cut into pieces
- 2 onions, sliced
- 2 carrots, sliced
- 1 cup mushrooms, sliced
- 1/2 Tsp black pepper
- 1 tsp salt

Directions:

Add celery, onions, carrots, and mushrooms into the slow cooker.

Place chicken over the vegetables.

Combine together wine, water, red pepper flakes, pepper, and salt and pour over the chicken.

Sprinkle with parsley and basil.

Cover slow cooker and cook on high for 4 hours.

Serve and enjoy.

Nutritional Value (Amount per Serving):

Calories 258

Fat 8.5 g

Carbohydrates 6.5 g

Sugar 2.9 g

Protein 33.8 g

Cholesterol 101 mg

93-3 Ingredients Chicken Tacos

Total Time: 6 hours 10 minutes

Serving Size: 6

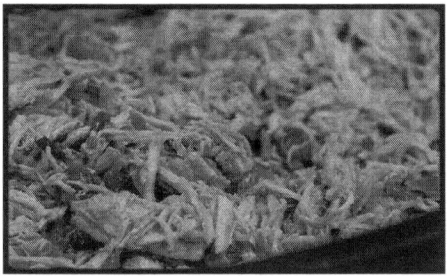

Ingredients:

- 1 1/2 lbs chicken breasts, skinless and boneless
- 1 packet taco seasoning
- 14 oz tomatoes, diced

Directions:

Place chicken into the slow cooker.

Sprinkle taco seasoning over chicken.

Add diced tomatoes into the slow cooker.

Cover slow cooker and cook on low for 6 hours.

Using fork shred the chicken and serves.

Nutritional Value (Amount per Serving):

Calories 234

Fat 8.5 g

Carbohydrates 3.9 g

Sugar 2.1 g

Protein 33.4 g

Cholesterol 101 mg

94-Delicious Ranch Chicken

Total Time: 4 hours 5 minutes

Serving Size: 6

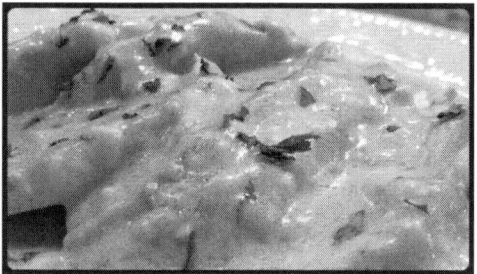

Ingredients:

- 2 lbs chicken breasts, boneless
- 3 tbsp ranch dressing mix
- 4 oz cream cheese
- 3 tbsp butter

Directions:

Place chicken into the slow cooker.

Add cream cheese and butter over the chicken.

Sprinkle ranch seasoning over the chicken.

Cover slow cooker and cook on high for 4 hours.

Using fork shred the chicken and serves.

Nutritional Value (Amount per Serving):

Calories 406

Fat 23.6 g

Carbohydrates 0.9 g

Sugar 0.2 g

Protein 45.3 g

Cholesterol 171 mg

95-Cilantro Lime Chicken Tacos

Total Time: 4 hours 10 minutes

Serving Size: 8

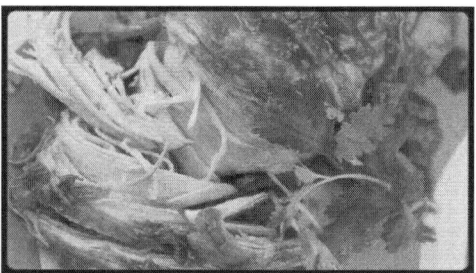

Ingredients:

- 2 lbs chicken breasts, skinless and boneless
- 2 lime juice
- 1/3 cup fresh cilantro, chopped
- 16 oz salsa
- 1 packet taco seasoning

Directions:

Place chicken into the slow cooker.

Add remaining ingredients over the chicken.

Cover slow cooker and cook on high for 4 hours.

Using fork shred the chicken and serves.

Nutritional Value (Amount per Serving):

Calories 236

Fat 8.5 g

Carbohydrates 4.9 g

Sugar 1.9 g

Protein 33.7 g

Cholesterol 101 mg

96-Yummy Chicken Carnitas

Total Time: 4 hours 10minutes

Serving Size: 10

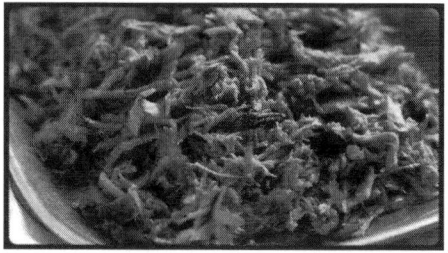

Ingredients:

- 2 1/2 lbs chicken breasts, skinless and boneless
- 1/4 cup cilantro, chopped
- 3 tbsp fresh lime juice
- 1 tbsp chili powder
- 1 tbsp garlic, minced
- 1 1/2 Tsp cumin powder
- 1/2 Tsp salt

Directions:

Place chicken into the slow cooker.

Add remaining ingredients over the chicken.

Cover slow cooker and cook on high for 4 hours.

Using fork shred the chicken and serves.

Nutritional Value (Amount per Serving):

Calories 221

Fat 8.6 g

Carbohydrates 0.9 g

Sugar 0.1 g

Protein 33 g

Cholesterol 101 mg

97-Roasted Herb Chicken

Total Time: 4 hours 10 minutes

Serving Size: 6

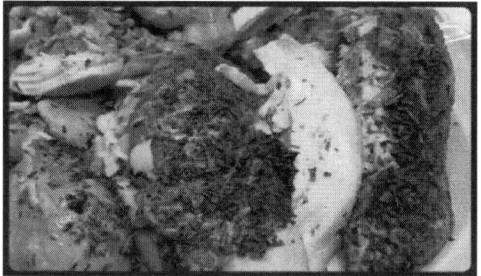

Ingredients:

- 3 lbs whole chicken, remove giblets
- 1 onion, sliced
- 1 fresh rosemary sprig
- 2 tbsp fresh thyme
- 1/2 cup fresh parsley, chopped
- 1/4 cup olive oil
- Pepper
- Salt

Directions:

Add olive oil, rosemary, thyme and parsley into the food processor and process until smooth.

Season chicken with pepper and salt.

Rub herb paste over the chicken.

Add sliced onion into the slow cooker then place chicken over the onion.

Cover slow cooker and cook on high for 4 hours or until chicken cooked.

Serve and enjoy.

Nutritional Value (Amount per Serving):

Calories 515

Fat 25.3 g

Carbohydrates 2.6 g

Sugar 0.8 g

Protein 66 g

Cholesterol 202 mg

98-Basil Thyme Chicken

Total Time: 4 hours 10 minutes

Serving Size: 6

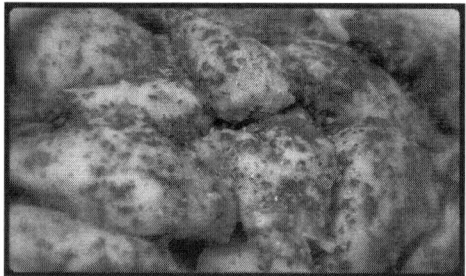

Ingredients:

- 2 lbs chicken thighs, skinless and boneless
- 1 tbsp fresh thyme
- 1 garlic clove, minced
- 1 tbsp fresh basil, minced
- 2 tbsp fresh oregano, minced
- 1 onion, sliced
- Pepper
- Salt

Directions:

Season chicken with pepper and salt.

Add chicken, thyme, garlic, basil, and oregano into the large zip-lock bag and place in refrigerator for 1 hour.

Place onion slices into the slow cooker.

Now add marinated chicken into the slow cooker.

Cover slow cooker with lid and cook on high for 4 hours.

Serve and enjoy.

Nutritional Value (Amount per Serving):

Calories 301

Fat 11.4 g

Carbohydrates 3.2 g

Sugar 0.9 g

Protein 44.2 g

Cholesterol 135 mg

99-Buttery Lemon Parsley Chicken

Total Time: 3 hours 10 minutes

Serving Size: 8

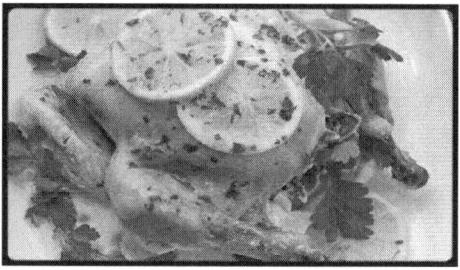

Ingredients:

- 5 lbs whole chicken
- 2 tbsp fresh parsley, chopped
- 4 tbsp butter
- 1 lemon, sliced
- 1 cup water
- 1/4 Tsp black pepper
- 1/2 Tsp kosher salt

Directions:

Season chicken with pepper and salt.

Place chicken into the slow cooker then pours water over the chicken.

Cover and cook on high for 3 hours.

Melt butter in a pan over medium heat.

Add parsley and sliced lemon into the pan and stir well.

Place cooked chicken on serving dish then pour butter mixture over the chicken.

Serve and enjoy.

Nutritional Value (Amount per Serving):

Calories 592

Fat 26.8 g

Carbohydrates 0.8 g

Sugar 0.2 g

Protein 82.2 g

Cholesterol 268 mg

100-Perfect Shredded Chicken

Total Time: 6 hours 10 minutes

Serving Size: 4

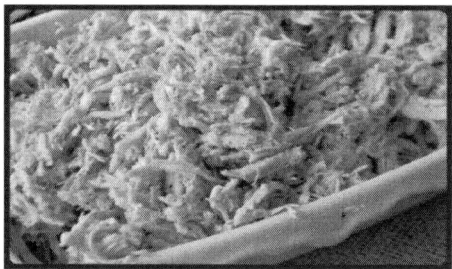

Ingredients:

- 16 oz chicken breasts, skinless and boneless
- 1/2 Tsp dried oregano
- 1 tsp onion powder
- 1 tsp garlic powder
- 1/2 cup chicken stock
- 1/2 Tsp black pepper
- 1 tsp salt

Directions:

Season chicken with pepper and salt.

Place chicken into the slow cooker.

Sprinkle oregano, garlic powder, and onion powder over the chicken.

Pour chicken stock into the slow cooker.

Cover slow cooker and cook on low for 6 hours.

Shred the chicken using a fork.

Serve and enjoy.

Nutritional Value (Amount per Serving):

Calories 222

Fat 8.5 g

Carbohydrates 1.4 g

Sugar 0.5 g

Protein 33.1 g

Cholesterol 101 mg

Printed in Great Britain
by Amazon